# WHEN THE DIAGNOSIS IS
# MULTIPLE SCLEROSIS

# WHEN THE DIAGNOSIS IS MULTIPLE SCLEROSIS

*Help, Hope, and Insights from an Affected Physician*

## KYM ORSETTI FURNEY, M.D.

The Johns Hopkins University Press
Baltimore

**Note to the Reader.** This book is not meant to substitute for medical care of people with multiple sclerosis, and treatment should not be based solely on its contents. Instead, treatment must be developed in a dialogue between the individual and his or her physician.

*Drug dosage.* The author and publisher have made reasonable efforts to determine that the selection and dosage of drugs discussed in this text conform to the practices of the general medical community. The medications described do not necessarily have specific approval by the U.S. Food and Drug Administration for use in the diseases and dosages for which they are recommended. In view of ongoing research, changes in governmental regulations, and the constant flow of information relating to drug therapy and drug reactions, the reader is urged to check the package insert of each drug for any change in indications and dosage and for warnings and precautions. This is particularly important when the recommended agent is a new and/or infrequently used drug.

First edition published in 2008 by Praeger Publishers, Westport, Connecticut
Johns Hopkins Paperback edition published 2009
9 8 7 6 5 4 3 2 1

The Johns Hopkins University Press
2715 North Charles Street
Baltimore, Maryland 21218-4363
www.press.jhu.edu

Library of Congress Control Number: 2009922915

ISBN 13: 978-0-8018-9392-6
ISBN 10: 0-8018-9392-5

A catalog record for this book is available from the British Library.

*When the Diagnosis Is Multiple Sclerosis: Help, Hope, and Insights from an Affected Physician* by Kym Orsetti Furney, M.D., was originally published in hard cover by Praeger Publishers, an imprint of Greenwood Publishing Group, Inc., Westport, CT. Copyright © 2008 by Kym Orsetti Furney. Paperback edition by arrangement with Greenwood Publishing Group, Inc. All rights reserved.

*Special discounts are available for bulk purchases of this book. For more information, please contact Special Sales at 410-516-6936 or specialsales@press.jhu.edu.*

The Johns Hopkins University Press uses environmentally friendly book materials, including recycled text paper that is composed of at least 30 percent post-consumer waste, whenever possible. All of our book papers are acid-free, and our jackets and covers are printed on paper with recycled content.

*When life gives you lemons, make lemonade . . .*

A poster with these inspirational words hung on my bedroom wall throughout my adolescent years. With the naiveté of a child, I had assumed the phrase meant that I should make the most of the gifts I was given. In recent years, I saw that phrase emerge again. As an adult I realized that, of course, the lemons represented some sort of misfortune that should be transformed into something good. I laughed at myself for my innocent interpretation for all those years. Somehow, I now see this book as representing a product of both of my interpretations of those lemons.

# CONTENTS

# PREFACE

*"Multiple Sclerosis." What a terrible disease. This can't be right. Not me. Not now. I'm busy. I have a daughter, a husband, a job. How can I possibly go on?*

I chose to write this book because I have never forgotten the flood of frightening thoughts and emotions that I experienced when I was diagnosed with multiple sclerosis (MS). I am hopeful that by sharing some of my experiences, your own path may be made a little easier as you either face a new diagnosis of MS or struggle with some of the challenges that arise during the first few years.

Being diagnosed with relapsing–remitting multiple sclerosis came as a tremendous shock to my whole sense of self. At age 34, I considered myself to be healthy and fit, and I was at a wonderful point in my family life and career. I had a bubbly, little fifteen-month-old daughter, and I was thinking about having another child. I had studied long and hard to finally be working as a physician of internal medicine. My husband and I were learning how to balance two careers while maintaining a strong sense of family. Then, one day, very unexpectedly, I began to feel lightheaded whenever I was standing. Next came the spinning sensation. Within a week, the diagnosis of multiple sclerosis caused the walls of my very happy life to come crashing down.

It has been seven years since I was "officially" diagnosed with MS and thirteen years since I had optic neuritis, often an early indicator of future MS. Fortunately, I still consider myself to be healthy and fit. I now have two daughters, a great part-time job, and a husband who continues to be a tremendous source of strength. I still exercise, help to coach my daughter's soccer team, and enjoy life to the fullest. And, yes, I regularly inject myself with medication because I do have MS. Yet, I can say with complete honesty that I do not feel like the MS has me. While some days are more challenging than others, I do not believe that my life has been dramatically altered because I live with MS. Most important, I have learned how to maintain hope for the future.

My path to reaching a point where I can make such statements included many difficult experiences. As I encountered various challenges along the way, I sometimes wished that I had a way to tell others with MS what I had learned in going through a particular situation. Eventually, I started writing down some of these thoughts, and I am glad to be sharing them with you now.

I am hopeful that my perspective as someone who is both a patient and a physician will allow me to have a better connection with you as a reader while still "getting the facts straight." Most often in writing this book, I share my thoughts as a person who has struggled with a decision or situation that arose because of my MS. As I do so, you will come to know that you are not alone in experiencing the spectrum of overwhelming emotions that may sometimes come with these challenges. Occasionally, I put on my "doctor's hat" and convey some pieces of advice that come from the in-depth reading I have done about multiple sclerosis because of my own illness. In sharing this dual patient-physician perspective, it is my hope that you will finish this book with some new ideas, attitudes, and understanding about living with MS.

One of the biggest challenges for me in writing this book was the realization that there will never be a "one size fits all" book for everyone living with MS. Multiple sclerosis is an illness that affects each individual in a slightly different way given its great variety of potential symptoms. In addition, we come from many different backgrounds, in many different colors, and speak many different languages. Therefore, no two people living with MS are likely to have identical symptoms or challenges. As you read, it may be helpful to keep in mind that we are all different. Yet, I am fairly certain that over time, there are many common emotions and situations that we encounter.

Since I do not want the main text of this book to be too technical or full of medical jargon, I am including an "appendix" that provides some of the more technical information that you may want to know about MS. It is important to realize that I am writing this book as someone living with the relapsing–remitting form of multiple sclerosis (RRMS). The appendix defines exactly what it means to have RRMS and also explains the other types of multiple sclerosis.

If you are newly diagnosed with multiple sclerosis, you may want to start by reading the first four chapters. The titles of the subsequent chapters are self-explanatory and you will know when you are ready or have the need to read them. For others who are further along in living with MS, you may choose to flip back and forth between chapters as various situations arise.

My overriding message to you is one of hope. As you can see from the chapter titles, there are clearly going to be some bumps in the road. In sharing my thoughts, I wish to make some of those bumps a little smoother. While it may take some time to come to terms with the diagnosis of MS, I do believe that you will come to a point where your outlook is positive and your life feels complete again.

# Acknowledgments

My greatest thanks goes to my husband, Scott. The only reason I found time to write this book is because he created that time for me by taking our children on countless expeditions to the park, pool, and other fun places. His support throughout the process was never-ending, even when my computer was seeing so much more of me than he was. As I have dealt with my MS over the years, he has been my sounding board and my source of strength.

Next, I thank my mother, whose proofreading of each chapter likely saved me from multiple rewrites for my publisher. I now understand and appreciate why she took so much time to teach me how to write when I was in elementary school.

I thank both my mother and my father for their gentle guidance and direction over the years. Their continuous support and faith in me has kept me going during the most challenging of times. My sister, Kathy, who lives a courageous life with cerebral palsy and a smile on her face, reminds me what life is all about.

My girls, who are now eight and five years old, had very little direct involvement in the creation of this book. Yet, they were always patient and understanding when I told them it would only be a few more months until mommy had her book written and could join them on the fun expeditions with daddy. In addition to my husband, they are the light of my life. Their giggles and hugs make life worth living.

I thank all of my close girlfriends who never seemed to tire of my talking about my book and my concerns about getting it done on time. I thank Susan Dorr Goold, M.D., who may not realize that she played a pivotal role in the first week of my diagnosis by being that person who *really* understood what I was going through. I thank Cicley Worrell Sullivan, whose example of optimism and courage showed me how much more I could be doing within the MS community.

Thank you to Dr. Michael Kaufman, a brilliant neurologist who brings an incredible amount of time, genuine care, and critical thought to each patient he sees. And, thank you to the National Multiple Sclerosis Society for helping me to see myself in a much more positive light.

# 1

## BEING DIAGNOSED

### THE NAME, "MULTIPLE SCLEROSIS"

I have a very hard time with the name of this illness—"multiple sclerosis." It has such a horrific sound to it. Even after seven years, I rarely say the words *multiple sclerosis* aloud. I much prefer the more appealing sound of *MS*. In speaking to others with multiple sclerosis (MS), I have learned that I am not alone with this preference.

At the time I was diagnosed, I was somewhat familiar with this illness, having intermittently cared for multiple sclerosis patients in the hospital. Most of the patients I had seen were diagnosed with MS in the 1970s or 1980s, a time when medication for relapse prevention was not yet available. Others, who were frequently in the hospital, had a variant of MS called "primary progressive multiple sclerosis," which can lead to significant disability fairly quickly. As a physician, I thought their situations were so very sad, as many patients had developed poor functioning of their arms, legs, bladder, or speech. I rarely had the opportunity to see the MS patients who had very little disability, since they were seen in the outpatient setting. So when I finally had it confirmed, that yes, these bizarre symptoms I had been having were in fact due to multiple sclerosis, I conjured up the worst possible images of what might happen to me.

While many of you may not have had the opportunity to meet patients with more advanced stages of MS, I suspect that your reaction to the diagnosis of MS may have been quite similar to mine. Many people still carry an image of multiple sclerosis as an illness that picks an individual out of the prime of his or her life, and leaves that person wheelchair bound and severely disabled. Fortunately, for the majority of women and men who are newly diagnosed with relapsing–remitting MS in the new millennium, this is not an inevitable outcome. And yet, while we know that medications now exist to prevent relapses, this knowledge does not necessarily make the initial journey any easier. We did not sign up for this club. We did not ask to play this game. The anger, the grief, and the uncertainty about the future can be overwhelming.

Give yourself time. It will be possible to feel in control again.

## My Diagnosis Story

There are countless different symptoms of multiple sclerosis. Therefore, no two individuals will have exactly the same physical or emotional experiences. I share the account of my own diagnosis because hearing the stories of others' diagnoses was so helpful to me when I was newly diagnosed. Listening to others' stories made me feel as if maybe I could actually survive as a member of this club. Again, not a club that I would have chosen to sign up for, but a club that is full of understanding and support. The stories of others comforted me and made me feel less alone.

I share with you my entire diagnosis story, although somewhat long, because this is frequently the reality of being diagnosed with MS. It was six years from the time that my first symptoms appeared until I knew with certainty that I had MS.

I was twenty-seven years old, engaged to be married, and working long hours as a resident physician when I began to experience pain in my left eye. It felt as though I had pulled a muscle in my eye, but as a physician, I knew that was unlikely. I assumed the pain would be gone in a few days. Instead, the pain increased. I began to have difficulty driving because of the pain brought on by looking to the extreme left or right. I decided to call a resident physician whom I knew in the Department of Ophthalmology, and he suggested that I be evaluated in clinic sometime that week. Two days later, I went for my appointment, where a different resident physician asked a lot of excellent questions and did a thorough eye exam. He could not see anything wrong with my eye but recommended "monitoring" the symptoms so that I could let him know if anything changed or got worse.

*As is the case for so many patients in the early stages of MS before a diagnosis has been made, I left the appointment feeling somewhat foolish.* I felt that I had wasted my own limited time as well as the time of the resident ophthalmologist. I attributed my symptoms to the stress of a busy inpatient rotation where I was caring for cancer patients in addition to the stress of preparing for a wedding. I left the office and returned to the hospital to tend to my patients who were truly sick as they battled various cancers. I again dismissed the eye pain since I now knew there was "nothing wrong."

A few days later, I was shopping for bridesmaid dresses when I began to sense that something was not quite right with my vision. I stopped in the middle of the store, looked straight ahead, and realized that I could not see the left side of the room. My stomach turned, and panic slowly set in. Now I was scared. While I still did not have a definite diagnosis in mind, I knew something had to be very wrong. The resident physician a few days earlier had asked, "Are you sure there are no changes or problems with your vision?" Well now there were problems. The thought of potentially losing my vision altogether nearly paralyzed me.

I paged the resident physician whom I had seen in the office, and I described my partial visual loss on the left, trying to sound calm and professional. His tone was now quite serious. Gone was his easy-going demeanor of a few days prior. He would see me with his supervising physician first thing in the morning. His level of concern only escalated my own fear. I did not ask him what he thought was wrong, and he, of course, was not going to tell me anything over the phone. At that point in my Internal Medicine training, I had never seen a patient with optic neuritis, the diagnosis I was soon to have. Therefore, I certainly did not know that optic neuritis can be an initial symptom of MS. So while I had trouble falling asleep the night before that appointment, I still did not know what was coming.

The next morning, within minutes of examining my eyes and hearing my symptoms, the supervising neuro-ophthalmologist sat down with me and told me I had "optic neuritis." In a manner that was much too straightforward for me as I was suddenly transforming from physician to patient, he told me that optic neuritis could be associated with multiple sclerosis. However, he went on, there were many instances when it occurred without having MS. I learned that I would need an MRI scan of my brain to visualize my optic nerves and to see if there was any indication of MS. As for my visual symptoms, I would *probably* recover most of my visual function. Oh, and if the MRI confirmed the optic neuritis, I would need to receive three days of high-dose intravenous steroids, starting as soon as possible, to help with my visual symptoms and perhaps to prevent the future onset of multiple sclerosis.

I choked back the tears with my stomach in knots as I tried to maintain my composure as the professional physician that I thought I was supposed to be. We were still sitting in the relative darkness of the eye examination room as the supervising physician provided this onslaught of information for me. To this day, what I remember most about that morning was that it all felt very *dark*.

The hours that followed that appointment are somewhat of a blur. I know that I called my fiancé first to tell him. He also did not know much about optic neuritis, so his initial response was very calm and supportive. I then had to arrange for coverage at work so that I could get my MRI done and begin receiving intravenous steroids. That night, my fiancé and I sat at my kitchen table, flipping through the pages of a medical textbook, trying to educate ourselves about this diagnosis of optic neuritis. Reading together, we came to the page where it said between 30 and 70 percent of patients with optic neuritis would go on to develop multiple sclerosis. All the strength that I had been mustering up was gone. "30 to 70 percent." Multiple sclerosis might truly be in my future. I started to weep. My fiancé held me and wept with me.

The MRI was done within twenty-four hours, and there was wonderful news to be had. The scan did not show any definite signs of MS. However, both the left and right optic nerves were involved, even though I only had symptoms on the left side. The following morning, instead of putting on my white doctor's coat, I found myself feeling like a foreigner in uncertain territory as I lay on a stretcher in a hospital gown, having an IV catheter poked into my arm. Once the IV was in place, explanations followed from a nurse about what to expect as the steroids were infusing—perhaps a metallic taste in my mouth, perhaps some heat and flushing. My fiancé by my side and holding my hand, I was glad to be doing the right thing for my health. The tears of forty-eight hours earlier were gone, and I was back in my "pull-it-together Kym" mindset. *Denial* had already begun to settle in as I protected myself from my worst fears. My MRI showed no signs of multiple sclerosis. I did not have MS, and I was not planning on getting it. The optic neuritis had just managed to sneak in during a stressful time of my life.

Thirteen years later, as I look back to my episode of optic neuritis, perhaps I was fortunate in that it gave me a chance to contemplate the possibility of having MS without having to receive the actual diagnosis. Unlike the experience of many other MS patients, I was also fortunate in that it was only days from my initial eye symptoms until I had some definite diagnosis. I did not have to endure months or years of different doctors and different symptoms, wondering what was wrong with me or if I was just crazy.

For me, my vision recovered nearly completely within weeks of treatment, and life went on. And on it went quite well. I got married, finished my residency training, began working as an Internal Medicine physician and gave birth to a beautiful little girl. I was happy and busy, so I rarely thought about the possibility of MS. A neurologist had once said to me that if I made it five years from my initial optic neuritis diagnosis without any new symptoms, I would probably never have MS. Even though I spent little time thinking about the possibility, I do distinctly remember making a mental note to myself in April 1999 when I was seven months pregnant with my first child, that those five years had passed without any apparent symptoms.

One morning, fifteen months after the birth of my daughter, I was supervising resident physicians in a very busy outpatient clinic. I began to notice that I felt lightheaded whenever I stood up from the discussion table to go to a patient's room. Within hours, this dizzy sensation had become persistent, and I had to put my head down on the table just to tolerate the sensation. I excused myself from the supervising room and asked a nurse to check my blood pressure. My pressure was surprisingly low and my heart rate was abnormally fast. I began to think of all the things that could be causing my symptoms—blood loss, dehydration, a thyroid problem, perhaps a second pregnancy. However, I had no reason to have any of those problems and had not yet made the decision to have a second child. Despite having had optic neuritis six years earlier, the diagnosis of multiple sclerosis did not even cross my mind that day. *Denial can be surprisingly strong.*

Being a physician admittedly allows for rapid access to other physicians. Within three days, I had seen a neurologist and a cardiologist. Both of these

very intelligent doctors thought I had a form of "postural orthostatic hypoten-
sion" that can sometimes be seen in young women without a definite cause.
The neurologist did not think I needed to worry about MS, and an MRI was
not ordered.

Two nights later, I got up to use the bathroom at three o'clock in the
morning. On my way back to bed, I was struck by profound dizziness and
spinning. I fell to the floor. It felt as though the floor were a magnet, pulling
my head back down and preventing me from getting back up. I called my
husband's name. His strong arms carried me back to bed, where everything in
the room continued to spin even though I was lying perfectly still. Did I have a
brain tumor, was I bleeding inside my head? Although terrified, I still did not
realize that a diagnosis of multiple sclerosis was twenty-four hours away.

Needless to say, this spinning episode greatly concerned the neurologist I
had seen a few days prior. That evening, I found myself back inside the tight
space of the MRI machine. With my head wedged tightly between foam blocks
and cage-like bars inches from my nose, I thought of my daughter sleeping
soundly in her crib at home. If this were to be MS, would I be her soccer coach
someday, would I walk down the aisle at her wedding? A hot tear trickled
from the outer corner of my eye, flowing down my cheek and onto my neck.
The loud, clanking sounds of the MRI scanner continued. I prayed as my heart
raced.

I tried to see my own patients in the office the following day to keep my
mind off the fact that I was anxiously awaiting the results of the MRI scan. The
day slowly crept by, and at 4.30 P.M., I still had not received a call from the
neurologist. My husband and I could not wait any longer. As I went in to see my
last patient, my husband went over to the radiology department to find the
results. I had just stepped out of my patient's room to get some information
sheets when he returned. The look on his face told me the news, but I still
had to hear the words from him to be sure. *Yes, it was MS.* Queasiness filled
my stomach as I felt the walls closing in. Somehow, I kept my composure long
enough to return to my patient's room to give her the necessary papers and
answer a few more questions. My husband was waiting for me as I came out.
We grabbed our coats and walked in silence ever so quickly to our car, as if
we were trying to escape an evil that was chasing us. As soon as we were both
inside the car and I slammed the door shut, the sobs came uncontrollably in a
way I had never experienced before. My husband held my shaking body.

# 2

## GRIEVING

I have promised to deliver a book about hope, yet I have begun with some very powerful feelings of sadness. Certainly not everyone will experience this emotion to the extent that I did. However, I suspect that almost everyone who faces a new diagnosis of multiple sclerosis feels some degree of sadness. If you are going to come to terms with the diagnosis and be able to move forward, I believe it is extremely important that you allow yourself to experience this feeling rather than to deny that the sadness exists.

For most, the sadness is accompanied by some sense of loss of who you are. You, as you have always perceived yourself, have somehow changed. Your body has betrayed you, allowing things to happen without your permission. Even if you are fortunate enough not to have acquired any permanent physical disability at the time of your diagnosis, you have taken on a new, emotional burden. Many of you who are newly diagnosed with MS may be like I was at the time—relatively young, in good health, and not in need of chronic, daily medications. A diagnosis of multiple sclerosis completely changes that self-perception. There will be injection medications on a regular basis, and perhaps additional medications to deal with the symptoms of MS. When you fill out a health form, you will no longer be able to circle all the No's.

For the first few weeks after my diagnosis, I went about my daily business very aware of myself as "a person with multiple sclerosis." I *labeled* myself, and in doing so, it affected how I thought I was supposed to function. Even though my physical abilities returned to the same level they had been several weeks prior, I felt as though I was suddenly supposed to be less capable. I briefly questioned whether I would be able to continue my job or to be a good mother. Not surprisingly, after thirty-four years of living with a very positive attitude, this changing self-perception made if extremely difficult for me to maintain my upbeat outlook.

Very aware of my own sadness, I tried to identify all the good things about the situation. Thank God this was not the brain tumor that I had pondered weeks before as I lay in bed with the room spinning. This was not a terminal diagnosis. I was not going to die from this. Yet, despite these efforts at looking for the brighter side during the first few months, the darker side still found a way in. No, this was not a death sentence, but it was a sentence for life. I was not going to be able to make it go away.

While I certainly would not discourage you from trying this strategy of looking for the positive aspects of your situation, I believe it is just as important to acknowledge the true feelings you are experiencing. One of my intentions is to reaffirm for you how perfectly normal it is to feel sad, overwhelmed, and perhaps even hopeless at the time of diagnosis. It is very appropriate to *grieve*. Allowing yourself the time to grieve will likely provide you with greater mental health in the long run.

What exactly do I mean when I say we should allow ourselves to grieve? Typically, we think of grieving as a process that a person goes through when he or she has lost a loved one. In the medical profession, we also refer to the grieving process for a patient who has been given a terminal diagnosis. When diagnosed with MS, we may be grieving for a lost sense of self. We may be grieving as we anticipate a lifelong diagnosis that is likely to present many challenges along the way. The actual process of grieving will be somewhat different for each of us. While we share a common diagnosis, each of us is a unique individual. We will move from a grieving phase to a point of acceptance at different speeds and in different ways.

## STAGES OF GRIEF

As you may know, a woman named Dr. Elisabeth Kubler-Ross spent a great part of her life researching and writing about the five stages of grief[1] for those who have been given a terminal diagnosis. The stages she describes include denial, anger, depression, bargaining, and acceptance. I do not believe that every person necessarily goes through each of these stages in this order. Nor do I want to overemphasize the grieving process with a diagnosis of MS because we have not in fact been given a terminal diagnosis. However, if we are aware of these stages, we may recognize some of the same emotions in ourselves. In doing so, we are again reassured that this is a normal process and are reminded that we are not likely to feel this way indefinitely.

If you are someone who had unexplained symptoms for many years prior to your diagnosis of MS, you may not experience significant feelings of denial. There may actually be a feeling of relief to finally have an explanation for the years of symptoms. However, if you were diagnosed fairly quickly and unexpectedly, your sense of denial may be very strong. Even though I was a physician who had experienced an episode of optic neuritis in the past, I still felt a sense of shock and denial when multiple sclerosis was confirmed on my MRI.

In living with MS, I believe that a mild degree of ongoing denial may always be occurring and is likely to be helpful for us. We cannot live every minute of every day with the diagnosis of MS at the forefront of our minds. If we did, we might not allow ourselves to live our lives to our fullest capabilities. For the most part, I now go about my daily routine without thinking about the fact that I have MS. I do not think about my MS as I am seeing patients throughout the day at work, or as I am playing with my children in the backyard. Certainly, there are moments each day when my chronic arm or leg numbness may become worse that I am reminded about my MS. There is the obvious reminder whenever it is time for my injection medication. However, most of the time, my MS "sits on the back burner" as I go about my day.

While a small amount of denial can be a very effective coping mechanism, it is important to distinguish this from a complete sense of denial that prevents an individual from ever accepting his or her diagnosis. A young woman whom I met recently was diagnosed with MS two years ago at age 19. While she had acknowledged the importance of the disease by being very active in MS fundraising activities, she had not taken ownership of the disease process as something that was actually occurring within her own body. After a brief attempt at using an injection medication, which resulted in adverse effects, she completely stopped taking her medicines. Because she feels well now and has not developed any physical disability, she believes that she does not need any medication at this point in time. This is an example of denial preventing someone from pursuing different medication options that might be better tolerated and might maintain her health for the long term.

For me, the anger that I felt about my diagnosis was very short-lived. When Dr. Kubler-Ross described a stage of anger, she was referring to a sense of "this isn't fair" or "why me?" As a physician, I have seen enough terrible illness to believe that no one gets through life without some burden of suffering at some point in time. Even outside of the hospital, I have watched friends and colleagues face great personal challenges. During the same year in which I was diagnosed, my closest friend suddenly lost her father in a tragic accident, another friend struggled with repeated miscarriages, and another had a child born with a severe disability. Prior to my diagnosis, I was very aware that I lived an extremely fortunate and healthy life. As I was diagnosed, I realized that multiple sclerosis would be the personal challenge that I was going to have to confront. Although I still struggled greatly with the diagnosis, I never felt terribly angry.

While anger did not play a large part in my personal grieving process, your experience may be quite different. If you are overwhelmed with anger and feeling that your situation is simply not fair, it is certainly normal to feel that way. Many people with MS initially feel a strong sense of injustice when they are diagnosed. *Why am I the only one I know having to deal with this for the rest of my life?* Allowing yourself to experience the anger at the beginning, rather than to suppress it, may eventually enable you to feel ready to let go of some of those feelings. As with denial, you may never completely let go of every bit of the anger. However, with time, those feelings should diminish to a point where you can move toward acceptance.

The bargaining stage for someone who is facing a terminal diagnosis is described with thoughts such as, "I promise I will be a better person if this disease could just be cured and I am allowed to live." Because we are very fortunate not to be facing a terminal diagnosis, our initial bargaining may be a little different. "I promise to be a better person if I can just not have any more relapses." While I may not have those precise thoughts, there is a different kind of bargaining I do somewhat subconsciously as I live with MS. I tell myself that if I take my medications faithfully, exercise regularly to the extent that my body allows, and eat as well as I can, then my MS "should behave and stay quiet." Of course, these are all the right things I should be doing to modify the disease process anyway. Therefore, this version of bargaining can work in our best interest. However, this is healthy only as long as we recognize the reality that there are no guarantees in this bargaining process. Relapses are still likely to occur at some point in time. Nonetheless, our overall health should be better for having a sense of doing our part.

Depression, another one of the stages of grief, is a topic that deserves a chapter all to itself later in this book since it can occur anytime during the years that we live with MS. However, feelings of sadness early on are an expected part of the grieving process as we come to accept our diagnosis of MS. My personal sadness was quite profound in the first few weeks following my diagnosis. The depression was a very complex process for me as it involved my feelings of decreasing self-worth and changing self-perception, as well as a sense of guilt in letting down those who depend upon me. I felt the full impact of the diagnosis whenever I envisioned how it might affect my life in the future. I cried a lot when I was alone, and I cried as I repeatedly shared my fears with my husband. Fortunately, over the weeks, my feelings of sadness and despair started to lift. I had talked to many friends and family. My husband and I had many discussions about our future together. I started to feel like I needed to do something. It was time to move on.

If your feelings of sadness persist for months after your diagnosis, and you do not begin to feel the weight of depression lifting, then you should share these feelings with your physician. It is normal to feel sad for a period of time as a reaction to a difficult diagnosis. Physicians may sometimes refer to this as "situational depression." However, if weeks turn into months and you are still experiencing extreme sadness or despair, then your neurologist or primary care physician may suggest treatment for what may then be referred to as "clinical depression." With clinical depression, many aspects of your behavior and health may be affected, including changes in your appetite, your sleep habits, or your ability to think clearly and concentrate. Treating clinical depression with an antidepressant can result in significant improvement in these symptoms.

## SUPPORT FROM OTHERS

As we move through the stages of grief in our own unique ways, support from others is absolutely critical. The burden of these emotions should be shared. Simply having another person who cares about us to act as a sounding board can provide much needed comfort. Many loved ones or friends may feel somewhat uncomfortable because they "don't know what to say." Letting them know that you just want someone to listen may allow them to feel more comfortable in their role. I was extremely fortunate to have a husband who listened with great patience. Beyond that, I also gained an immense calming effect from talking to a colleague at work who had been diagnosed with MS one year earlier. While my husband was a wonderful listener, there was no way for him to truly know how I was feeling. My colleague knew first-hand what I was experiencing. I did not need to explain. She had passed through the grieving. Her life seemed "back to normal." She allowed me to see that I would get to that point too.

Beyond family and friends, there are now many great MS support groups to help us get through the tough times or just the everyday times. If you are still in the early stages of diagnosis and are having a difficult time coming to terms with your diagnosis, you should not hesitate to seek out one of these groups. Talking to another person with MS can be invaluable. Even someone who is initially a stranger will soon be a close ally as you share your experiences. Your local chapter of the National MS Society or the support group from the pharmaceutical company that manufactures your injection medication are both good places to start if you are seeking some additional support. (See the "appendix" for Web sites and phone numbers.)

## ACCEPTANCE

Not everyone who is diagnosed with MS or any other illness necessarily passes through each of the stages of grief. It is important to realize that these stages are not always clearly defined or recognizable for the person who is experiencing the emotions at the time. I chose to discuss the stages of grief because it is through grieving that we come closer to some degree of acceptance about our diagnosis. Acceptance is what positions us in a place where we are ready to take care of our body, mind, and spirit.

In closing this chapter, I want to share two important caveats about grieving and acceptance:

1. We should never expect to be completely and entirely finished with the grieving process and to say that we are never coming back again. At some point in the future, there are likely to be relapses of our MS. Or, we may have weeks that are exasperating for other reasons and we get frustrated that we have to deal with MS on top of life's other stressors. During these times, we may again briefly dip into feelings of anger, bargaining,

or depression. But, if we are otherwise doing well with our emotional health, these should be brief stops along the way. When the stops are not brief and the negative feelings become persistent, it is time to seek assistance.

2. I have emphasized the importance of accepting the diagnosis of multiple sclerosis. By that, I mean that we should be able to say to ourselves, "Yes, I have multiple sclerosis." We need to be willing to learn about the disease in order to keep ourselves healthy. We need to be ready to take the recommended medications and to see our doctors regularly. However, acceptance does not mean that we feel happy about having MS, or that we even feel completely at ease with the diagnosis. I certainly accept the fact that I have MS. However, if given the opportunity not to have it, of course I would take that opportunity. So I have accepted having multiple sclerosis so that I might take all the necessary steps to keep the disease at bay. By taking an active role in the management of my disease, I am able to maintain hope for the future.

# 3

# THE PSYCHOLOGICAL CHALLENGES OF MS

The previous chapter on grieving focused on many of the emotional challenges that come with a diagnosis of multiple sclerosis. However, the challenges referred to within the title of this chapter are somewhat different. Many of us who are recently diagnosed with MS are fortunate to have only mild physical disability or minimal symptoms. So why then does this diagnosis result in such an overwhelming reaction? The answer for most of us is that there is an incredible fear of what the disease might take away from us over time.

Not knowing the future course of our own disease process is, in my opinion, one of the greatest long-term psychological challenges of living with MS. Because of the lack of predictability of multiple sclerosis, we must live with uncertainty. If we are going to experience a relapse, we have no idea when it might occur. We cannot choose to schedule a relapse for a time that might be more convenient in our lives. We also cannot choose from a menu what type of symptoms we might experience with a relapse. Because the symptoms of MS are so varied, we may also frequently wonder whether some new symptom is in fact a result of our MS. All these factors can feed into a feeling of lack of control over our disease. These are the ongoing psychological challenges of living with MS.

## WHAT DOES MY FUTURE LOOK LIKE?

"Am I going to be in a wheelchair someday?" Whether we voice this concern aloud or not, this is a common fear of many who are diagnosed with multiple sclerosis. While the medications currently available make it less likely that those with a new diagnosis of relapsing–remitting MS will find themselves in a wheelchair at some point, there are never any guarantees. There is no fortune-teller with a crystal ball who can tell us what our future holds. In reality, I think *not* being able to predict the future course of our MS is extremely beneficial to both our mental and physical health. A fortune that told us we will be without disability in twenty-five years might cause us to grow lazy in our good habits or might allow us to believe we could skip our medications. On the other hand, a fortune that told us we will be using a wheelchair in twenty-five years would likely cause despair in the present, even when our situation is still quite good. We might not want to play an active role in our disease management, feeling there was no reason to do so. Therefore, we must try to find a way to appreciate that the uncertainty about our future is what encourages us to develop healthy habits and to participate in the management of our disease. Most important, by not knowing what the future holds, we are able to maintain a sense of hope.

As I encourage an attitude of hopefulness in living with MS, there are definitely times when I do worry about the future. It remains very difficult for me to watch those with MS who were diagnosed twenty-five years ago when medications were not yet available. As I watch someone struggle with the simple task of pouring a cup of coffee, or the challenge of maneuvering a motorized scooter, I want to look away. I am afraid. I don't want that to be me someday. I don't want to see how MS can take away a person's basic abilities. In many ways, I feel like a coward compared to those with disabilities whose incredible inner strength keeps them going. Yet, I know my reaction is normal. So rather than continuing to worry, I allow a small amount of healthy denial to creep back in. I remind myself that I am an MS patient in an era of medications to treat the disease. Therefore, it is reasonable to hope that my outcome may be better because of the medications.

## COULD THIS BE A SYMPTOM OF MY MS?

While most of us will reach a place where we do not worry about the distant future all the time, there may be more frequent psychological challenges brought on by various symptoms that we may have. Prior to my MS diagnosis, I never thought much about feeling a little dizzy if I got up from bed too fast, and I did not worry if I still felt tired after a good night's sleep. However, during the first year after my diagnosis, I would worry that every little twinge or temporary feeling of numbness was going to be a relapse. Even though I was a physician and I might be able to come up with another explanation for a particular symptom, I still worried.

The symptoms of multiple sclerosis are varied and can occur in many different parts of the body. This aspect of MS greatly adds to the challenge of living with the disease. As patients, we must attempt to interpret the array of symptoms we may experience. This is in contrast to a patient with asthma, for example, who knows that he is likely having an exacerbation if he begins to feel more short of breath or begins to wheeze or cough more. Asthma and many other chronic illnesses have a better-defined set of symptoms. It is difficult for a neurologist to provide us with a complete list of symptoms that might indicate an MS flare. When we are shown a list of potential symptoms of

MS, this may unintentionally provoke more anxiety. We might begin to worry about which symptoms we will have in the future. Or, we may realize that many of the symptoms are not unique to MS and might occur when we simply catch a cold.

During the seven years since my diagnosis, the psychological challenge of worrying about various symptoms I experience has become much less burdensome. Now, if I have been sitting with my legs crossed for half an hour and I cannot feel my foot afterward, I do not panic. I know that my foot has "fallen asleep" from having my legs crossed, and the feeling will come back in a few minutes. I have also learned that while I would want to report any new symptoms of a potential relapse to my neurologist fairly quickly, there is rarely going to be an MS symptom that is a medical emergency requiring treatment within the next hour. So when I do experience a symptom that I am not sure how to interpret, I usually wait twelve to twenty-four hours before I decide if I need to call my neurologist. During that window of time, it usually becomes clear to me whether the symptom is something to take seriously. If the symptom is completely gone within twenty-four hours, it is very unlikely that an MS relapse is taking place. If the symptom persists or gets worse, then I know it is time to make a phone call.

I certainly do not want to underestimate the importance of letting our neurologists know when we are worried about a potential relapse. Some relapse symptoms will be obvious and waiting to call the neurologist would not make sense. (For example, your leg becomes extremely weak, or you are so dizzy that you are having difficulty standing.) However, the variable symptoms of MS will have us wondering many times whether a new feeling or symptom is related to our disease. As you gain experience with your own body and this diagnosis, you will have a better sense of when a symptom deserves rapid attention. Over time, a sense of panic will not set in every time your leg falls asleep or you feel a little out of sorts when a cold is coming on.

## A Friend's Story . . .

I became friendly with a thirty-one-year-old woman at an MS fundraiser a few years ago. At the time I met her, it had only been a few months since she was diagnosed with MS. Her diagnosis had been made when she developed symptoms of weakness and numbness in her leg, making it very difficult for her to walk. Fortunately, she had recovered complete use of her leg and appeared healthy and physically fit. At the fundraiser, I was very impressed with her positive attitude and proactive position, particularly given the newness of her diagnosis.

My new friend and I had met for lunch on one or two occasions after the fundraiser and had been communicating by e-mail about an upcoming MS walk in which we were going to participate. Then, one evening, she called me at home. I initially thought she was calling with an update about the walk.

However, within a few seconds, I knew that something was wrong. The usual perk and strength of her voice were absent. She told me she had just been out to dinner with her boyfriend, but had to leave the restaurant because she just did not feel right. She "felt funny in her head." I temporarily switched from my friend role to my doctor role and started to ask her some specific questions about her symptoms. As she described to me what she was experiencing, her tears came. This very strong woman was confronting one of the psychological challenges of living with MS. She was extremely worried that her symptoms represented a relapse of her MS. Knowing exactly what she was feeling, I had to work hard to prevent my own tears from coming.

On the phone, she went on to tell me that she had been on a trip two days before and was not well rested. She had also been on an antibiotic for several days for a sinus infection. I suggested that both of these factors could be contributing to her current symptoms. I told her that I, being her friend and not a neurologist, could certainly not guarantee her that these symptoms were not due to MS. I did offer her reassurance that a good night's sleep might make a big difference. I let her know that it was very reasonable to wait until the next morning to see how she felt before she called her neurologist. I shared with her all the times during the past six years that I had been in her situation, wondering if a symptom was due to my MS. I let her know that she was not crazy for being scared. I listened, and she knew that she was not alone.

My girlfriend caught up on her sleep, talked to her doctor, and stopped her antibiotic. Ten days later, we walked together in the MS fundraiser. She felt completely well and had not had a relapse.

## LETTING GO OF THE WORRIES . . .

Yes, I still worry about the future of my health. And yes, I certainly have symptoms that scare me from time to time. However, for the most part, I am now at a place with my MS where I focus on staying healthy. I have decided that spending a lot of emotional time and energy worrying about the future of my MS would be a waste of that valuable time and energy. Worrying about it is not going to change whatever the eventual outcome may be. I know that I am taking my medication and doing what I can to stay well.

A reader of this book who is newly facing a diagnosis of MS may think, "Good for you and all your positive talk, but I don't feel like being so upbeat right now." It is important to understand that getting to the point where I am now took a long time. It has been seven years since my "official" diagnosis and thirteen years since my episode of optic neuritis. It took almost eighteen months following my diagnosis before I felt that I was truly myself again. It took that length of time to realize that the diagnosis did not need to define who I am. It took time to realize that I could actually have some sense of control of my life again. It took time to look at the world in a positive light again.

I am also the first to admit that, by not having had a major relapse in several years, my positive outlook is much more readily maintained. (I still knock on wood along with a prayer as I write this.) While I have episodic worsening of chronic symptoms such as arm and leg numbness or eye pain from time to time, I have not recently had to confront a major set of new symptoms in the form of a true relapse. If I had been having relapses and major symptoms every three to six months during the past seven years, I cannot be certain that my outlook would be as good as it presently is.

Initially, I hesitated to discuss the fortunate course that my disease has taken since the time of my diagnosis. My MS has responded quite well to the medications. This will not necessarily be true for everyone who is newly diagnosed with relapsing–remitting MS. Yet, there is no doubt that I do have multiple sclerosis. The MRI of my brain shows several white lesions on it that are classic for MS. However, I share the course my MS has taken because it is a key component in my desire to provide you with optimism for your own future.

I know that MS can sneak up on me when I least expect it, but I no longer live each day worrying about it. I try to live each day to the fullest with all the capacities I currently have. Should those capacities change at some point, I know I will face a difficult period of readjustment. For the time being, I try to live each day with hope.

# 4

# FACING THE NEEDLE: THE MS MEDICATIONS

A sudden change of topic to the potentially intimidating subject of injection medication may seem somewhat abrupt. Yet, while some of the emotional stages are going to take time to work through, it is very likely that you are immediately facing the challenge of self-injection. Neurologists usually recommend initiation of medication as soon as a diagnosis of multiple sclerosis is made in order to slow down the accumulation of new lesions and, perhaps, to slow down the development of disabilities. Therefore, your doctor probably does not want you to take the next three months to become comfortable with the idea of giving yourself a shot. If you have not already done so, you will want to gain confidence with the injection process fairly soon. Acquiring that confidence involves learning the technical skills needed for the injection process as well as overcoming the psychological challenge of sticking oneself with a needle.

## ISN'T THERE ANOTHER OPTION?

Your initial reaction to information about injection medication probably included thoughts that were similar to mine. "Injection, do they mean a shot? There must be a pill I can take. I can't possibly stick myself with a needle on a regular basis." This is one more component of the initial-good-news-followed-by-bad-news MS roller coaster ride. While there may be substantial relief in hearing that there are excellent medications to decrease the frequency of relapses, it can be disheartening for us to learn that the medications come only in an injectable form.

Even as a physician who has familiarity with handling needles at work, I still had a sense of dread about self-injection. After all, the needles I use at work are never pointing in my direction. In many ways, I felt additional pressure to do the injections as if I were comfortable with it simply because

I am in the health care profession. I imagined that everyone thought, "She's a physician. She can handle it, no problem." Yet, it does not matter who you are or what you do for a living. Shots hurt. Fear of a needle is a normal human reaction. We all learned at a very early age to dislike injections as we went for our annual childhood checkups and received our immunizations So, not surprisingly, for many patients with newly diagnosed MS, the idea of regular self-injection presents itself as a frightening and almost insurmountable task.

I am the first to admit that if I could pop a pill every day instead of self-injecting, I might think that managing my MS is a breeze. There is something about receiving an uncomfortable injection at least several times per week that in itself makes this disease seem more burdensome. To those looking in from the outside, a logical response might be, "Oh, come on, what's a little needle to help keep your MS under control? You are so fortunate to have an effective medication to take." Yet, for some of us, these frequent injections are a trying experience.

The process can be unnerving for the obvious reason that we are being asked to do something to ourselves that goes against our natural instincts. For me, the most difficult aspect of self-injection that I had to learn to tolerate was the actual discomfort of the needle breaking the skin. Whether you choose to use an auto-injector device or a prefilled syringe, there will always be the sharp sensation of the needle. For unclear reasons, my perception of that sharpness can change from one injection to the next. There are truly many days when I think, "Oh, that was easy, I barely felt that at all." Yet on other days, the needle may feel quite uncomfortable. It has become clear to me that different places on my skin have different sensitivities. For example, the middle of my abdomen is much more sensitive than my lower abdomen. My outer thighs tolerate the needle much better than anywhere else. During the first several times that you do your injection, realize that not every injection will feel the same. You may find areas that are just too sensitive to be used in the future. You will find other areas that will be your "good spots." Because it is important to rotate sites, you will eventually have your own "map" of your body to be used for injections that may look slightly different than the diagram that comes with your medication.

You may be thinking, "You have just increased my fear of self-injection by talking about sharp needles. I am losing confidence rather than gaining it." I realize that discussing needles may be an odd way to begin a chapter whose intent is to help you feel better about mastering self-injection. It is my hope that by confronting the worst aspect of self-injection up front, we can move on to discuss methods to overcome this fear of the needle. As you read, please keep in mind that the injection process does not come easily to anyone at first. Just as time will help with the emotional reaction to your diagnosis, time and practice will also help tremendously with the injection process.

## Removing the Psychological Barrier

One of the first steps in overcoming the psychological barrier to injecting yourself is changing your attitude about the injection. This is, of course, easier said than done. While the needle itself may never become your friend, the medication definitely will. When I first started taking my injection therapy, I certainly did not see the medication as my friend, and I wish someone had shared this perspective with me from the beginning. It has now been thirteen years since my diagnosis of optic neuritis, and I still exercise regularly as well as run, ice skate, and ski with my children. I still do these things because of my medication. The medicine is on my side. While it may take some time to see it this way, we are so very fortunate to have been diagnosed at a time when there is medication available to decrease the number and frequency of relapses. I am fairly certain that if you ask anyone living with MS who was diagnosed twenty-five years ago, that person would have been thrilled to have a good treatment option, even if it came in the form of a great big needle. In this current era of MS treatment, we have to overcome the relatively small challenge of self-injection to reap the potentially tremendous reward of staying well. The shot is so very worth it, and in the big picture of life's challenges, the shot can start to seem like less of an ordeal.

Are there days when I want to skip my injection? Absolutely. Interestingly, however, because I have done so well on the medication, I have now developed something close to a psychological dependency on it. At one point several months ago, there was a glitch with the mail order pharmacy from which I receive my medication, and there was going to be a two-week delay before I had my medication. Surprisingly, I felt a slight sense of panic. *But I need my medication, you don't understand, it keeps me well. I can't wait two weeks.* I quickly looked into ways I could get the medication through my local pharmacy and still have it covered by my prescription insurance. As you know, without insurance coverage, these medications are extremely expensive. Of course, my insurance would not cover it through my local pharmacy because they were already picking up the tab for the mail order, even though the shipment would be delayed. In the end, my neurologist was able to provide me with samples until my medication arrived. He also reminded me that panic was not necessary. A week without medication would be unlikely to suddenly increase my chance for a relapse after having been on the medication for so long. So while I cannot say that I actually enjoy the needle, I have come to value my medication tremendously.

## Practical Aspects of Self-Injection

You should never feel alone as you learn to self-inject. There are now countless resources to help you through the learning process. Most neurologists have experienced nurses working in their offices who will teach you initially.

In addition, all of the pharmaceutical companies that manufacture the current medications for relapsing–remitting MS provide a multitude of options to assist you as you learn. Most of the companies will provide a free, in-home nurse visit at your request. Some of the medication-specific web sites also have video clips demonstrating the injection process. Many neurologists' offices also have these videos available for loan to you. Lastly, all of the pharmaceutical companies provide toll-free phone numbers with live nurse support for any questions you may have about self-injection, medication side effects or other concerns. All the information you need about accessing the telephone or nurse support is readily available on the medication-specific Web sites. If you have computer access, I strongly encourage you to take some time to explore the Web site for your particular medication. Not only do these Web sites provide information to assist you as you are just starting out, but they continue to provide updates about your medication, discuss ongoing research and provide a sense of an online support group.

There may be some of you who feel that you simply are not ready to take on self-injection, so a spouse or significant other may learn to do the injections for you. I believe this is a good alternative for those who feel overwhelmed by the thought of self-injection. I also know that as time passes, many of these same people (who are physically able) will eventually choose to do the injections for themselves. One young woman with MS whom I met was initially quite fearful of giving herself injections. For the first year after her diagnosis, her boyfriend of many years did the injections for her. They later broke off their relationship but remained friends, and he continued to come to her home for several months to do the injections. Eventually, she felt ready for the independence that self-injection allows, and she learned to do her own injections. She now uses the auto-injector and does her injections with great confidence. Her story is not unique. There are many who may need some time to get used to the idea of injection therapy before they feel ready to do the injections themselves.

Because I do my own injections, I am aware that I have developed a certain bias toward the idea of doing one's own injections. I do believe a sense of empowerment eventually comes with giving yourself the medication. In doing my own injection, I take an active role in controlling my MS. It gives me the feeling of injecting a powerful medication right at the disease. In addition, there are the technical aspects that I would no longer want anyone else to do. I know how I like to hold my skin and how to angle the needle to make it as smooth as possible. I have a system and a routine. I like having control.

While I emphasize some of the benefits that may come from doing your own injections, the most important message is that you get the medication, whether you inject it yourself or someone else does it for you. Either way, you will of course be taking an active role in managing your disease process. By the very nature of our disease, there will be some who are physically unable to do self-injection. In those cases, a spouse, relative, or friend can learn the technique through the same resources I described earlier. Even if you are physically able to do self-injection, there may be areas that are difficult to reach, such as the back of your arms, where it may be best to have someone else do the injection for you. Sometimes, you may just want to take a break from the process. Within the first three to six months of taking your medication, you will likely develop a good sense for whether self-injection is something you will be doing alone or with a partner.

The word *routine* is absolutely critical in allowing the injection process to run smoothly. By making the injection part of your daily routine, it will come to seem as commonplace as brushing your teeth every night. As you think about a time of day for injection that will best fit into your routine, choose a time when the process will not feel rushed and when you are not likely to be interrupted. I have two young children who have no idea what it means for mommy to have privacy in the bathroom. Therefore, I choose to do my injections at night after they have gone to bed. If you are someone who hits snooze several times each morning and then rushes to get ready for your day ahead, then mornings may not be ideal for you. If you and your doctor have chosen a once-weekly medication, it might be best to choose a day of the week when the following day can be relatively restful. Once you select the time and days of the week that are best for your personal schedule, make an effort to stick with that general time frame on your injection days. This is what truly enables the process to become part of your routine.

In addition to choosing the time of day for your injection, it is important to create some protected space where you will keep your medications and supplies. Even if you are on a medication that remains refrigerated, having a space for your other supplies can be very helpful. I have a large drawer in one of my bathroom cabinets that contains only my injection supplies. I have chosen this location because this is where I do the injections. I have read about others with multiples sclerosis who have purchased storage containers or who have even made their own special boxes. Included in these supplies, I strongly encourage you to have a notebook to log the date and the actual location of the injection. Logging the site each time is the only way I can reliably rotate my injection sites. In the front of my notebook, I have written out the order in which I rotate the sites (e.g., left lateral thigh, right lateral thigh, right outside belly, left outside belly, etcetera). This tells me the location where I am due to give my next shot. It prevents me from favoring the spots that are easiest to reach or the least painful. Writing down the date of each injection also ensures that I never skip a dose. Life can get busy enough for all of us that we may not be absolutely sure if we are due for an injection that we may take three times a week, every other night or daily. If you are on a once-per-week injection schedule, the date may not be so important, but logging the injection site is still very important.

Figuring out exactly how you will rotate your injection sites is also something that will take a little planning. A pamphlet should come with whichever medication you take, showing a "map" of possible injection sites. It is important to try to use as many of these sites as you are able. However, also realize that in time and with experience, you may find that there are some sites that simply will not work for you. I tried the back of my arms many times but eventually gave up. It was very awkward positioning for me, and I did not like having visible injection site reactions when I wore short-sleeved clothing. Others I know use their arms on a regular basis. You will learn what works best for you. The injection sites suggested on the medication pamphlet are meant as a guide, not as an absolute set of rules. The medication will still be effective if you do not use every single recommended site. What is important is that you rotate your sites regularly, use as many sites as possible, and avoid using a favorite or easy spot too often.

## MEDICATION SIDE EFFECTS

One of the more common side effects that can accompany injection therapy is an effect frequently referred to as an "injection site reaction." If you have already begun self-injection, you may be familiar with this reaction. You may experience a burning sensation as the medication is going in, or you may be left with a burning or throbbing pain for several minutes after the injection. Depending on the medication you take and your own body's reaction to it, you may also be left with various lumps and bumps under your skin for several days following the injection. If you have any of these side effects, you may find yourself wondering if you are allergic to the medication or if your reaction is abnormal. You may also wonder why this is happening if you have never had such a reaction to previous shots throughout your lifetime.

Fortunately, most of these injection site reactions do not indicate an allergy to the medication. The reactions are due to the unique nature of the actual MS medications. While the medications may be very useful in controlling multiple sclerosis, our skin and underlying tissues are not so crazy about them. The reaction is more of a localized inflammatory process than a true allergic reaction. Of course, if you develop hives, prolonged itching, or other concerning symptoms, you should always speak with your doctor. Your doctor's office will be very familiar with the questions and concerns that come with injection site reactions. Do not ever hesitate to call them as you are newly navigating your way through the injection process.

I realize that the information provided about injection site reactions is not likely to be producing my desired effect of making you feel more comfortable with self-injection. The good news is that, for most patients, the severity of the pain and the extent of the skin reaction will lessen over time. While I can definitely report a decreasing level of discomfort over the years, I am still bothered enough by the reaction that I need to do something to soothe my skin. While each person's solution to alleviating the discomfort of injection site reactions may be slightly different, I will share some of the solutions that have been effective for me.

## SIMPLE SOLUTIONS

During the first three to six months of my current injection therapy, I had fairly severe pain at the injection site immediately following the shot. Therefore, I began to take a dose of ibuprofen approximately half an hour before the injection. While this did not eliminate the postinjection pain completely, it definitely seemed to lessen the severity. For a period of time, I also took a dose of an antihistamine such as diphenhydramine before I did the injection since some aspects of the injection reaction (such as a big red welt) do resemble an allergic reaction. Again, whether you use a pain-relieving medication, such as ibuprofen or acetaminophen, or an antihistamine before your injection is something you should discuss with your physician, but there are several options available.

The other remedy that I simply could not do without is the use of an icepack *immediately* after I inject. I have been doing this for six years now and believe it is a safe, inexpensive, and effective treatment for injection site reactions. I have been able to find some flexible, wallet-size icepacks that are just the right size. I keep one close at hand as I do my injection. As soon as the needle comes out, I apply the icepack to the area. I then wrap an ace bandage around the icepack and whatever part of my body I have just injected. This allows me to be up and about so I do not need to sit and hold an icepack on the injection site. There has been some debate over what a safe duration of icing time should be. Usually, five to ten minutes of icing should be enough to get the discomfort calmed down. There is concern that regular icing for periods longer than ten minutes might eventually lead to some skin or soft tissue breakdown. As an alternative to icing *after* injection, other resources suggest that icing *before* the injections can help. I have tried both ways and clearly prefer icing afterward. It is certainly worth trying both techniques if you experience painful injection site reactions to find the best solution for you.

## COMMUNICATING WITH YOUR HEALTH CARE PROVIDER

I share my own technique for dealing with injection site reactions because it is one of the more common side effects and can occur with the interferon drugs (Betaseron, Avonex, and Rebif) as well as with glatirimer acetate (Copaxone). For those of you who experience additional or different types of side effects that you feel may be coming from the medication, it is very important to communicate these effects with your physician or nurse. As with the simple solution of icing for injection site reactions, there may be other "quick fixes" for different side effects. For example, the flu-like symptoms of muscle or joint aches that may initially be present with the interferon drugs can be significantly decreased by taking medications such as ibuprofen or naproxen. It is also important to keep in mind that many of the side effects truly do diminish over time. And yes, there are many individuals who tolerate their medication very well from the beginning without any side effects. Less commonly, side effects may be so intolerable that you need to try a different medication altogether. Good communication between you and your health care provider will enable you to find the solutions and the medication that work best for you.

I worry that sometimes patients may feel like they are a "bad patient" if they "complain" too much about the difficulty they are having with a particular medication. In living with MS, we will require a lifetime of treatment to manage our disease. Therefore, finding a good fit with our medication is the only way we are likely to stay with our treatment program for the duration. I am on my third MS medication during the seven years that I have known about my diagnosis. Each of those changes occurred because I spoke up about particular concerns or side effects. When I voiced my concerns, I was a patient describing very real problems. I was not a physician quoting some statistic. I am now extremely happy with the quality of life I have on my current medication, and I feel that I could stay on it indefinitely if my MS continues to be well controlled with it.

## CHOICE OF MEDICATION

The medication you take will certainly be based in large part on the recommendation from your treating neurologist. Currently, there are six medications approved for use in relapsing–remitting MS. The particular medication recommended for you is likely to be based on a number of factors. At any given point in time, a new study may have just been released about one of the drugs, leading your neurologist to a particular choice. The specific symptoms that you experience with your MS or other underlying medical problems that you may have can also influence the choice of medication. Lifestyle issues may also play an important role in terms of the frequency with which the medication must be injected. This is where your input as a patient may assist your neurologist in making the medication decision. For example, someone who travels frequently for a job may prefer the weekly medication that is delivered as an intramuscular injection. Others may prefer a more frequent injection so that a subcutaneous injection can be performed. (See medication list below.)

The six drugs approved by the Food and Drug Administration (FDA) for the treatment of relapsing–remitting MS are usually referred to by the medical community as "disease-modifying" drugs. This terminology is used because currently there is no "cure" for relapsing–remitting MS in the way that most of us think of a cure for a disease. It is unlikely that a person taking these medications will never have another relapse. The medications will also not lessen any current symptoms that are a result of a prior relapse. However, there is an excellent chance that the medications will decrease the number of relapses you have in the future as well as decrease the number of new brain lesions accumulated over time. In accomplishing this, there should be a slowing down of the progression of disability over time. These are extremely important reasons to take a medication from the very start of your diagnosis.

Interestingly, recent studies have shown that individuals who do not even have a definite diagnosis of MS but have a neurological illness such as optic neuritis that can suggest future MS will prolong the time until they are actually diagnosed by taking some of these medications. If you are reading this book, you are likely already sure of the diagnosis. The point in sharing the result of those studies is to demonstrate "the sooner the better" effect in taking these medications. Putting off the start of medication until you have had a number of relapses or you are starting to have some disability is allowing the disease to get a jump start that you could have delayed or prevented.

The following is a list of the currently approved medications for relapsing forms of multiple sclerosis. For the most updated description of approved uses, dosing, and description of potential side effects, I would recommend viewing the Web site for each individual drug. If you are already on a particular medication, the material provided with the medication is usually very comprehensive.

*Interferon beta-1b (generic name)/Betaseron (brand name)*
Manufactured by Berlex Laboratories, Inc.
Approved for relapsing forms of MS
Given by subcutaneous injection every other day
Web site: www.betaseron.com
Nurse help line: 1-800-788-1467

*Interferon beta-1a (generic name)/Avonex (brand name)*
Manufactured by Biogen Idec
Approved for relapsing forms of MS
Given by intramuscular injection once per week
Web site: www.avonex.com
Support line: 1-800-456-2255

*Interferon beta-1a (generic name)/Rebif (brand name)*
Manufactured by Serono, Inc.
Approved for relapsing forms of MS
Given by subcutaneous injection 3 times per week
Web site: www.rebif.com
Support line: 1-877-447-3243

*Glatiramer Acetate (generic name)/Copaxone (brand name)*
Manufactured by TEVA Neuroscience, Inc.
Approved for relapsing–remitting MS
Given by subcutaneous injection daily
Web site: www.copaxone.com
Support line: 1-800-887-8100

*Mitoxantrone (generic name)/Novantrone (brand name)*
Manufactured by Serono, Inc.
Approved for worsening relapsing–remitting MS and for progressive–
    relapsing or secondary-progressive MS
Given by intravenous infusion in a medical facility up to 4 times per year.
Web site: www.novantrone.com
Support line: 1-877-447-3243


*Natazulimab (generic name)/Tysabri (brand name)*
Manufactured by Biogen Idec & Elan Pharmaceuticals
Approved for relapsing forms of MS.
Given by intravenous infusion at a medical facility monthly
Requires enrollment in a restricted prescribing program and regular moni-
    toring.
Web site: www.tysabri.com
Support line: 1-800-456-2255

## WHY WE DO THIS

It is hard for me to think about sticking myself with a needle on a regular
basis for the rest of my life. Just like anyone else doing injection therapy,
I remain hopeful that a pill will be developed that will be just as effective
or even better than our current medications. Such hope is not false. Several
good medications for MS that would come in a pill form are under active
investigation. However, we certainly cannot wait for these. The time to take
an active role in the management of our MS is from the very beginning. I
was shocked to learn that between my "clean" MRI in 1994 when I had optic
neuritis but no other brain lesions and the MRI when I was diagnosed in
2000, I had developed six new brain lesions. I never felt those lesions. I had
not experienced any perceptible relapses. I was fortunate that those lesions
occurred in areas of the brain that do not have much function. Nevertheless,
the disease process had been busy during those six years that I was not taking
medication. MS is not just about relapses. It is also about a silent attack on our
nervous system of which we may be completely unaware.

The medications *are on our side*, whether in the form of an injection, an
intravenous infusion, or a pill. I encourage you to do whatever it takes to get
started with your medication and to find the one that is best for you. Seek
out a support group, talk to your neurologist, talk to the trained nurses on the
other end of the help lines. In the long run, you will be physically and mentally
stronger because of it.

*Note:* For a more detailed discussion of the medications, please refer to the appendix.

# 5

# WHOM DO I TELL AND WHEN?

I have heard others with MS use the phrase "coming out of the closet" when they refer to telling others about their diagnosis of MS. This implies that people with MS may choose to keep their diagnosis a secret for a period of time, or they may choose to tell only select people. Some of you may read this and wonder why you would not readily tell most of the people in your life about your diagnosis. You may feel that having the support and understanding of others is critical to your own success. Of course, this is true.

However, because multiple sclerosis still carries the image of a devastating disease for those who know little about it, there is the potential for feeling labeled with that stigma for the rest of your life. There is the risk that others may initially treat you as if you are no longer the same person you were before the diagnosis. When you think about your own reaction to your diagnosis, you may have immediately conjured up images of those who have been most severely affected by MS. When you tell others who may not know much about relapsing–remitting MS in the current medical era, they may also wonder if severe disability is in your near future.

One of the wonderful things we can accomplish in choosing to tell others about our MS is to provide the opportunity for some of those older, frightening images of relapsing–remitting MS to be changed. In sharing our own experiences with those who are unfamiliar with current therapies and prognosis, we can demonstrate the way in which we are able to live relatively normal lives. However, early on in our own diagnosis, many of us may not feel ready to be the "poster child" for multiple sclerosis. We may still feel very uncertain about our own futures. The time for telling others while simultaneously painting a positive picture may not come for months or years after our diagnosis. We may not want others to know we have MS until we truly believe for ourselves that the diagnosis does not define who we are.

Just whom should you tell and when should you tell them then? The answer to this question will be different for each one of you reading this book. While I would never try to provide an answer to this question for anyone, I chose to write about this subject because it is something that every one of us will start to think about at some point in time once we are diagnosed. Unfortunately, at the beginning, I really did not give much thought to which people I would tell and how I might tell them. I wish someone had told me within the first few days of my diagnosis to slow down before I went around telling people in fairly casual conversation that I had MS. Because I did not give much thought as to how I would tell others, I ended up having some minor regrets about the way in which I quickly and casually told others out my diagnosis. I would have preferred to show some restraint and to choose my words carefully so that the situations would have been more comfortable both for me and the people I was telling.

Of course, when we are still reeling with the emotions of a new diagnosis, we may not be in a frame of mind to think carefully about any of this. By the time you are reading a book about multiple sclerosis, it is likely that you have already shared your diagnosis with those to whom you are closest. If you are reading this chapter because there are other people in your life who do not yet know about your MS and you are considering telling them, perhaps my thoughts and experiences will allow you to do a better job than I did in selecting which people to tell and how to tell them. You may also gain some new perspective in understanding the reactions of those you choose to tell.

## TELLING YOUR FAMILY

There are many different people that we call family. We also have very different relationships with various family members. At the time of my diagnosis, my most immediate family included my husband and fifteen-month-old daughter. Therefore, my husband had been completely aware of my symptoms, medical evaluation, and eventual diagnosis. For some of you, it may have been your parents, a significant other, or a close sibling who was involved as you went through the diagnostic process. These individuals may have known about your diagnosis from the very beginning.

Others of you may have gone through your diagnostic evaluation without sharing the details with anyone. Or perhaps, your spouse or parents did not come to the appointment the day your doctor told you the actual diagnosis. Therefore, just about all of us who are newly diagnosed will go through the process of telling those family members who were not present at the time of diagnosis. For some of you, there will be an instantaneous, pick-up-the-telephone reaction to call certain family members to let them know what is going on. Others of you may experience some reluctance to tell family members right away because you may worry about the reactions of the people who love you.

One would think that our families should be the easiest group of people for us to tell about our diagnosis. We would hope to have their unconditional support. We should feel confident that they will still love us no matter what the future holds. I was fortunate to know that these things would be true with my family. Nevertheless, I could not help but worry about how my family would "handle my diagnosis." When you have family members that love and care about you, you may feel hesitant to provide news that may cause them sadness or may cause them great concern. Yet, knowing that you will be able to share some of the emotional burden with your family can provide tremendous relief. We very much need the support that comes from telling family members. It is for these different reasons that we may have mixed feelings as we pick up the phone to call our families.

I am someone who had a difficult time mustering up the courage to tell my parents about my MS. I have always been very close to my parents. I attribute many of my personal accomplishments to their love and support. I had also always been the daughter they did not have to worry much about. I had encountered good fortune in school, with my professional life, with my new family, and thus far, with my health. I was a grown up, thirty-four-year-old woman. I did not want to feel like I was creating new issues for them to worry about at this stage of my life.

My parents lived seven hundred miles away from me at the time I was diagnosed. This provided the opportunity for me to get myself calm enough to tell them about my diagnosis without sounding too distraught. They had not been aware of my recent symptoms of dizziness and the subsequent medical evaluation. The onset of my symptoms had all happened so quickly that I thought I would wait until I knew what was going on before I told them anything. I had not anticipated that I would be telling them that I had MS.

I do not remember exactly how long I waited from the time of my diagnosis until I called my parents, but I suspect it was only twenty-four to forty-eight hours. While my husband had seen all the tears, my mom heard a calm daughter reporting the facts like the physician I was trained to be. "Remember when I had optic neuritis six years ago? Well, it looks like it finally caught up with me, and I actually have MS now.... Yeah, I have been having problems with dizziness for a few days..." And so the conversation went. I never shed a tear on the phone and neither did my mother. As silly as it may have been, I felt that I had to be strong for her. I am sure she felt the same for me. Yet, I felt great relief in telling both my mother and my father and in hearing their words of love and encouragement.

## REACTIONS OF FAMILY MEMBERS OR SIGNIFICANT OTHERS

Which family members we choose to tell first about our MS and their subsequent reactions are going to depend to some degree on the stage of life we are in. When I initially had optic neuritis and my fiancé and I learned that MS was a future possibility, one of my own concerns was that I never wanted to be a burden for him in the future. I told him that he did not have to marry me. We could just wait and see what happened. I was very fortunate that the only reaction I got from him was unconditional love and support. At that point, our relationship was already on very solid ground. If he ever considered walking away, he never shared it with me.

If you are in the earlier stages of a relationship with someone, there may be the concern of placing stress on your relationship by disclosing your diagnosis. There may be the fear of losing that person. In those situations, it may be helpful to seek out a local National Multiple Sclerosis Society support group for newly diagnosed patients and attend some sessions together with your significant other. Or, consider having that person come to your next doctor's appointment. Learning more about the hopeful future of relapsing–remitting MS together as a couple may help to decrease fears for both of you. For those who are already in a long-term, committed relationship, doing these things together may be just as helpful for you as well.

Another possible reaction from those who love us is that of *denial* about our diagnosis. Just as some of us go through a denial process when we are diagnosed, our loved ones may do this for many of the same reasons that we do. One woman I met at a fundraiser had been seeing different doctors for several years for symptoms of severe fatigue and lack of energy. She had experienced some minor neurological symptoms as well, but she had never thought much of them. When a physician finally told her he thought she may have multiple sclerosis, her husband immediately wanted her to go to another doctor for a second opinion. He thought the physician must be wrong. He loved his wife and certainly did not want her to have MS. His own denial mechanisms had kicked in. While this woman was not glad to have been given a diagnosis of MS, she was relieved to know that there was an explanation for all the fatigue she had been experiencing. After they had two consecutive visits with an MS specialist who ultimately confirmed the diagnosis, her husband no longer asked for further opinions. He began to read about multiple sclerosis. He became her biggest supporter. Several years later, he still helps her with her medication injections on the days that she needs a break.

A single, young woman in her late twenties with MS told me how her mother became very overprotective during the first few months after her diagnosis. Her mother insisted on staying with her in her apartment during her initial weeks of treatment. At first, the young woman was glad to have her support, especially as she was learning to do her injection therapy. But by the third month, she was back to work and feeling pretty well. Her mother kept expressing doubts about whether she should still be working at all. It took about a year for the mother to see for herself and to come to understand that her daughter would be able to continue to work. Now, her mother apparently still checks in by phone each week, but she is letting her daughter live her life as an independent adult.

The stories of these two women remind us that our family members who love us are also going to go through various stages of coming to terms with our diagnosis. In the beginning, they will not know any more than we did about what to expect for our futures with a diagnosis of MS. Fear, retreat, denial, overprotection, and grief may come from family members at various points in time.

Once we have shared our diagnosis with family members and significant others, keeping open the lines of communication is so very important. They need to know we are doing okay if in fact we are. This can help to ease some of their fears. If we are not doing so well, sharing this with them may allow them to provide the emotional support that we need and to give them a sense of participation in our care. Pointing your family members to good resources you have come across will also increase their knowledge about what you are going through. With that knowledge, they can then develop their own sense of calm and control. Learning more about MS will also give them ideas on how best to help you.

As I said at the beginning of this chapter, we are all so very different in who we are and how we will tell others. Some of you may find it strange that I felt a slight reluctance to tell my parents. Many of you may have quickly picked up the telephone or drove to your family members' house within minutes of your diagnosis. The way in which we tell our family members will be more personal than the way in which we tell anyone else. I cannot at all suggest what will be best for you. I can only say that because we love these people so very much, it may be the most emotional telling that we do.

## TELLING YOUR CHILDREN

This is a section where I must openly confess that I have no experience from which to write since my children do not know yet that I have MS. However, I am keenly aware of the importance and sensitivity of this topic. Telling our children will also be done in a personal and unique manner depending on the ages of our children and, perhaps, on the state of our own health. As I currently write this chapter, my daughters are seven and four years old. My oldest daughter was only fifteen months old when I was diagnosed. Since my second child was born, I have not had any major relapses that would be visible to them. They cannot see the numbness in my arm and leg, or the intermittent pain in my eyes. Most mothers of seven- and four-year-old children experience some fatigue, so I am not unique in that way either.

I definitely plan to tell my children. I am anticipating that it will only be another one to two years before I tell my seven-year-old daughter. I know that my reluctance in telling my girls is similar to the concern that all parents with MS have when they tell their children. I want my children to feel confident that mommy will still be there for them when they need me. I want them to feel confident that this illness will not take me away from them. My older daughter is already a "worrywart," so I do not want her to have increased anxiety in her young life because of my diagnosis.

While MS will never define who I am, it is now one component of what makes up who I am. I work hard to teach my daughters to accept people for who they are, regardless of how different they may be. So, I would not want to hide something from my children that may help them to further understand that everyone in life has a little something different about them. In addition, if and when I do have significant relapses, I want them to already have had some understanding of that possibility. Just as with the adults who love us, providing knowledge to our children will decrease their fears as well.

One thing I have learned with my own daughters is that children only absorb as much information as they are developmentally ready to handle. When my grandmother died last year, my older daughter, who was almost seven, had so many challenging and abstract questions for me. She gave great thought to the subject of death and briefly worried about whether my grandmother was okay. A few months later, she stopped asking questions about it altogether. In contrast, my three-year-old had said, "So your grandmother is in heaven?" I said, "yes," and that was the end of the conversation.

I suspect that when I tell my children about my MS, it will be very much the same. They will ask the questions to which they need answers at the time. As they get older, the questions will likely change. Before I do tell them, I will also do a little preparation so I can have good answers to their questions. While I may have a good amount of medical knowledge about MS, I want to be able to answer their questions in a way that is appropriate for children. The National Multiple Sclerosis Society provides a wonderful newsletter, called "Keep S'myelin," for children whose family members are living with MS. I have already looked at it many times and know that it can be a great resource as you plan to tell your children.

## TELLING COWORKERS: TO TELL OR NOT TO TELL

Deciding which coworkers to tell and when to tell them may present the greatest dilemma as you disclose your diagnosis to various people over the years. If you work outside the home, there may be an immediate need to figure out what you are going to tell coworkers at the time of your diagnosis. Some of you may be focusing more on the issue of whether or not you will be able to continue in your current job. (Please read more about this important issue in Chapter 6.) If you anticipate continuing in your current job but need to take some time off at the beginning, you may wonder what reasons you should give coworkers about why you will be out. By the time you are reading this, many of your initial decisions about what to tell your coworkers may have already been made. Since this is frequently an issue that has some urgency, we do not always have time to read a book or visit a Web site to provide some guidance in this decision-making process. Even if you have already made it through "round one" of telling certain coworkers, the issue of telling those at work about your diagnosis may come up many times through the years in your job, either as you switch jobs or as new coworkers come and go.

While we may have some concerns about emotional reactions from family members when we tell them about our diagnosis, telling colleagues at work may carry some risk. The biggest worry may be the possibility of losing our job after telling about our MS, even if we are physically and cognitively well enough to do our job. Unfortunately, there are many true stories in the MS literature that describe individuals who have encountered job loss after disclosing a diagnosis of multiple sclerosis. Even if we believe that job loss would be unlikely, would we suffer from discrimination and be less likely to get future promotions? Would coworkers suddenly see us as less capable? Even though there is legislation in place that protects us from discrimination in the workplace if we choose to disclose our diagnosis, we cannot change the natural reactions and feelings of coworkers and employers as they learn that we have MS.

When we think about coworkers who have taken time off for illness, it is frequently with the expectation that the person will be treated and return to work as his healthy and "normal" self again. If someone is out from work with pneumonia, it is reasonable to expect that person to return at some point in time and be "all better." The person may still be weak or tired for a few days, but he is not going to have pneumonia forever. Or, for those who face quite serious illnesses such as a cancer diagnosis, they may be gone from work for a prolonged period. Yet, when they return, we think of them as having been treated and on the road to recovery.

Once we tell coworkers we have MS, we cannot take it back. Even if we are fortunate enough to be able to tell them how well we are doing, we still have been labeled with a chronic illness. It will take some time after we have told them that we have MS to show them that we can still do our job. In the beginning, we may not be completely sure that we will be able to do all aspects of our job. We may need time for ourselves to see if our symptoms are going to resolve or improve. It is very possible that we make actually need to make some job modifications due to physical limitations, cognitive problems, or fatigue. But, until we feel we have reached our own understanding of how our disease is going to affect us, it may be wise to limit the number of coworkers we tell or the extent of what we choose to tell them.

This does not mean we should be lying to or deliberately misleading our colleagues. Trustworthiness is paramount to any job relationship. However, it is still quite truthful to tell your boss or coworker, "I am going to start some treatments for this dizziness I've been having. I'll know more in a few weeks about how well I am going to respond." Or, if your coworkers have been unaware of your symptoms, you may not need to reveal any details initially.

The decision to tell coworkers will depend, in part, on each of your unique job situations. Some of you may work in very small businesses or job environments where coworkers are like family. You may feel very comfortable in sharing your diagnosis with them. Others may work in large corporations where you choose to tell just a few close colleagues. For some of you, a visible physical disability at the time of diagnosis may make it necessary to provide at least some information about your situation. Yet even in that situation, you may choose to report that you are undergoing medical evaluation and hope to see some improvements in the near future. All of that would be true in the setting of relapsing–remitting MS.

Again, I would never encourage the deliberate deception of coworkers. Instead, I suggest giving yourself a little time to better understand the ways in which your symptoms of MS will impact the abilities that are required of you to perform your job. Then, if and when you choose to inform coworkers, you will be able to provide a more accurate picture of what a diagnosis of multiple sclerosis means for you at that point in time.

### Mistakes I Made

The thoughts I have written about telling colleagues at work seem very logical to me now, seven years later than the time I first did my telling. Unfortunately, as I look back, I realize that in being overcome with my emotions during the first week I was diagnosed, I gave no thought as to whom I would tell or how I might tell them.

I believe there is an aspect of human nature that gives us the desire to inform others around us when we have been hurt in some way. We expect the responses from other human beings to be supportive and to provide a touch of sympathy that may be needed. When a loved one dies, we tell those who are close to us so that we may have their support. When we are particularly sick, we let others know so that they might support us until we have recovered. These are the types of situations we are likely to quickly share with the coworkers we know fairly well. So perhaps I should not be so surprised that I found myself quickly divulging my diagnosis to coworkers within days of my diagnosis. Yet, without any forethought as to exactly what I might tell them, I caught some colleagues feeling very unprepared as I was suddenly telling them something of a fairly serious nature. Unfortunately, I clearly left some coworkers feeling uncomfortable and uncertain as to what to say.

The worst example of my "inappropriate telling" came within three days of my diagnosis. I found myself telling another physician colleague about my diagnosis in a little kitchenette where we would go to get coffee in the mornings. We were doing the usual morning exchanges when he said, "So what's new?" I did not hesitate to say, "Well, I am having a hard time this week because I was just diagnosed with MS." He felt terrible to hear the news, and of course he had very little to say because he never knew such serious subject matter was coming his way. Since my severe episode of dizziness had taken place at home, my milder symptoms of dizziness had not been visible to anyone at work. I realize that I was feeling hurt in some way and in need of support from others. Yet, blurting out my diagnosis to a colleague in front of the coffee machine was not the right way for me to go about telling others.

Fortunately, the circle of colleagues I told at work that first week was relatively small. Being in a job with physicians who are used to maintaining patient confidentiality, I did not worry about other coworkers' hearing my news "through the grapevine." Therefore, after those first few months of my diagnosis, I did have time to give more thought to whom I would tell and when. As I started to feel physically well again with the dizziness gone and the realization that I was still going to be me, I suddenly did not want everyone else at work to know about my MS. I did not want to be labeled. I did not want my colleagues wondering if I would be able to do my job. I decided that I would tell individual coworkers when the timing felt right. I also realized that there would be some coworkers that I would probably never tell.

### Keeping a Secret

Admittedly, to this day, I sometimes still feel like I am keeping some *really big secret* from coworkers or any others that I have chosen not to tell about my MS. Now, because I have been fortunate to do quite well with my medications and I feel good about my future, I am much more comfortable in being open about having multiple sclerosis. (Hopefully that is the case or I should not have written a book about living with MS!) Yet, I have also come to realize that just because we have MS, this does not mean that we have to be ready to wear the diagnosis on our sleeves. That will always be our personal choice.

Think about the coworkers you know. Are you aware of all of their chronic medical illnesses? Do you know who is treated for high blood pressure, diabetes, heart disease, or depression? Perhaps you do know for those colleagues to whom you are the closest. But do you believe that your coworkers must inform you if they are being treated for high blood pressure? You probably would not think this is necessary as long as their condition does not affect the way they can do their job. Therefore, you should not feel an obligation to tell coworkers about your diagnosis as long as you are physically and mentally capable of continuing with your job.

The issue of being physically and cognitively capable of doing our jobs is another very important topic. Certainly, the very nature of MS is such that we cannot predict whether we will always be able to perform our current job. Because we might worry about the need for our job description to change in future years, we may feel more of an obligation to inform coworkers at the present time. However, a person with high blood pressure or high cholesterol could also have a heart attack in the future, potentially changing his ability to do his job. Yet, we probably would not feel that people with these illnesses are obligated to tell coworkers. If you are well enough in the present to continue with your job, you can address future changes in your health status and the potential impact on your job if and when those changes occur.

Clearly, I have slanted my discussion about the decision to tell coworkers in a way that favors withholding information about your diagnosis. Some of you will quickly see yourselves as MS advocates and choose to be very vocal about telling others right away, including your coworkers. I applaud this choice and admit that it is a braver position than I had been able to take for many years.

Because of my own preconceived thoughts about MS that took a long time to change, I simply did not want to feel labeled. In addition, as a physician, I did not want to feel that the work I did was being critically judged because of my diagnosis.

Having said all of that, if those of us with relapsing–remitting MS who continue to work were to be open about our diagnosis, we would continue to shed a positive light on the changing image of RRMS. Others would come to know that in our current medical era, multiple sclerosis is not all about doom and gloom. They would see what great contributions those of us living with MS continue to make to society.

### My Approach

Yes, there are good reasons to be open about your MS at the workplace. There are several, equally good reasons to limit the coworkers you tell. There are no simple answers. It has taken me many years to feel comfortable in disclosing my MS diagnosis to anyone, and it took the longest to gain that comfort in telling coworkers. My current approach with colleagues at work is to give people a chance to know me for a period of time before I tell them about my diagnosis.

When I moved from the state where I was originally diagnosed to a new location several years ago, I knew that I would eventually choose to tell certain coworkers at my new job. However, I waited six to twelve months before I chose to tell this new group of colleagues. I wanted them to know me first as a person without any particular diagnosis. I wanted them to have seen what I was capable of doing in my role as a physician. When I did eventually choose to disclose my diagnosis to coworkers in the appropriate settings, there was always some surprise. However, my colleagues had already come to see that having MS had not prevented me from doing my job. They did not have the need to express any sympathy for my situation. Instead, I received many positive comments. Several times I heard, "That's great that you are doing so well." Even if they had thought about what the future held in terms of my job, I no longer worried that they might be thinking about it.

## TELLING FRIENDS

### Close Friends

Some of us have friends that feel just as close to us as our family does, and we will likely approach telling them in the same personal way we did our families. In the beginning, we want and need the unique kind of support that only a close friend can provide. Nevertheless, even with my closest girlfriends, I still struggled in deciding how best to tell them. Just as I had felt with my family, I did not want my girlfriends to feel saddened by my diagnosis. I wanted their support, but I did not want them to worry. As I told each one, their reactions were all similar. "I'm so sorry. What can I do to help?" I told them that the best thing they could do would be to listen during the times that I needed to talk.

Those girlfriends have been wonderful over the years. While I have been relatively fortunate with my MS, there are occasionally bad weeks when various life stressors lead to significant eye pain or extreme fatigue. These friends have always provided an ear to listen, a babysitter to watch the kids for an hour, or someone to bring dinner over after a long day at work. These relationships feel so comfortable that I do not hesitate to let these friends know what is going on with me. If you have friends like this in your life, sharing your diagnosis with them will likely lead to a lifetime of understanding and support.

## Social Friends

There is another layer of friends that come after those I have already described. For me, as a married, working mom, these social friends are the other moms I know from my children's schools, other couples with whom my husband and I attend social events, friends at church, and neighbors. If you are younger or single, these may be friends from school, work, or other social activities. We usually encounter these friends in social situations, and we frequently have fun and casual conversations with them.

When I was first diagnosed, I was not sure if I wanted to be open about my MS with this group of friends. I again worried about that vulnerable feeling I might have once I shared my diagnosis. I did not want these friends to treat me any differently than they had before they knew about my MS. I wanted to be sure they would still ask me to sign up to volunteer for the next school event. I wanted to be sure they would still ask me to go to the gym to work out as we had always done.

Just as with colleagues at work, I knew there were many good reasons to share my diagnosis with this circle of friends. These friends again provided me with the opportunity to shine a positive light on the face of multiple sclerosis. I could let them see all that I was still doing. I could educate them about the ups and downs of living with MS. For those times when I was feeling stretched with work, home life, or the kids' activities, I knew that having them aware of my situation would allow for some understanding when I felt that I simply could not volunteer for another activity.

Over the years, I have slowly told my "social friends" about my MS when the opportunity presented itself and the timing felt right. Despite my own concerns, I have never regretted telling them. I have been amazed at how supportive people can be without making me feel pitied. As a result of knowing about my diagnosis, many of these friends have also been more likely to participate in MS walks, bike rides, and other fundraisers without any prompting from me. It is an amazing tribute to the goodness of people in general and to those we call friends.

## EDUCATING OTHERS AS WE TELL THEM

As we make the decision to tell others, whether family, friends, or coworkers, there is an excellent chance that these individuals will have questions about our diagnosis. Some may be afraid to ask questions if they think that the answers may not be very happy ones. Therefore, I think it is helpful both to you and to those you tell to have some idea of what other information you want to provide besides the fact that you have multiple sclerosis. It is much less uncomfortable for those you tell if you can follow what may seem like bad news with some additional news that carries a positive message.

What that message will be is going to depend on each of our personal experiences with MS. Even though I am never in my physician role when I am telling someone about my diagnosis, I sometimes find myself providing that person with medical information about MS. I frequently tell others that there are different kinds of MS, and I have the kind called relapsing–remitting multiple sclerosis. I tell them I am fortunate because there are now good medications that I take to keep the disease under control. I let others know that I am certainly still at risk for relapses, but I take one day at a time. Providing this information can put others at ease, and it opens the door for them to ask questions if they have any.

When you are first diagnosed, you may not be ready to provide others with so much information about MS. It may still be hard just to say the words *multiple sclerosis* when you are talking about it in terms of yourself. When you are still feeling this way and find yourself telling family or friends about your diagnosis, it is much easier to say that you are still learning about MS and the treatments. You will know if and when you are ready to teach others about it.

## THE UPSIDE OF TELLING

While I have shared many of my personal concerns and challenges in disclosing my diagnosis of MS to certain groups of people, it is important for me to finish this chapter by emphasizing that I have never had any regrets about telling those whom I have over the years. While I may regret the hasty and awkward way that I told some people in the beginning, I never regretted that those people had the information. In fact, each time I tell another person, I feel a slight burden lifted. Revealing my diagnosis decreases my sense of living a double life, trying to keep track of those who know and those who do not. Each person I tell gains a more complete picture of who I am. Each person I tell is likely to be supportive and understanding. Each person I tell will come to understand why those of us with relapsing–remitting multiple sclerosis are able to feel hopeful about what the future holds for us.

# 6

# IMPACT ON OUR JOBS

"Will I still be able to do my job? *Should* I continue to do my job? Is the stress of my job going to affect my MS?" Whether you work at a desk job or have a physically demanding job, these questions are likely to cross your mind in the weeks following your diagnosis. As with all the issues in this book, the answers are going to be as unique as each one of us. Yet, there are common themes to these questions that we can all consider as we go forward in making career decisions.

Being diagnosed with multiple sclerosis came as a significant blow to my sense of self. It initially changed the way I thought about myself. But on the day I was diagnosed, I was still a wife, mother, and physician. These roles essentially defined who I was at that point in my life and they still do. Fortunately, the diagnosis did not suddenly cause me to be incapable of fulfilling those functions. So, it became very important that I make good decisions about how I would continue to perform each of these roles. Of course, my career as a physician was the role that had the greatest potential to change depending on the choices I made.

## AM I STILL PHYSICALLY AND MENTALLY CAPABLE OF DOING MY JOB?

There is something about being told we have multiple sclerosis that has the potential to make us feel like we are supposed to be less capable of doing the things we have always done. Of course, it may be appropriate to feel this way if we are in fact having physical or cognitive symptoms that may truly interfere with our line of work. Yet, we may still feel as if we are suddenly less capable even if our symptoms are not severe or are likely to be temporary. The older, debilitating image of MS in the premedication era may initially impact the way we think about what we will be able to do.

During the first few weeks after my diagnosis, I wondered, *Are there other doctors with MS who are working? My job is emotionally demanding and I spend a lot of time on my feet. Will I still be able to do this job?* Of course, in the first week, I was still experiencing significant dizziness and had a fairly numb leg. Those were just the physical problems. Emotionally, I was in no position to be making smart or rational decisions about my career.

It may be a few weeks or even months after your diagnosis before some clear answers begin to emerge about what will be the best approach to your job. As we know, symptoms from a first episode or an exacerbation that led to a diagnosis of MS may take several weeks to resolve or to come to a new baseline. The answer to whether you are physically and mentally capable of continuing to do your job will differ dramatically depending on the type of job you have and your specific symptoms. Those whose jobs involve heavy physical labor may find themselves feeling challenged to continue a job at the same level of exertion. An executive at a big corporation with a "desk job" may feel just as challenged if he or she is dealing with debilitating fatigue.

The good news is that there are thousands of people living with MS who work in the community and make meaningful contributions everyday. In addition, we now live in a society where people with disabilities from all different causes have a visible place in the workforce. Employers have become familiar with making adjustments for employees with disabilities. There is legislation called the "Americans with Disabilities Act" (ADA) that requires employers to make "reasonable accommodation" for such employees. Of course, interpretation of what may be considered a reasonable accommodation has the potential to become complicated. My simple goal for someone who is new to these types of issues is to make you aware that the ADA exists. Employers in our country are generally well aware of it. (If and when you are ready to learn more about this, I refer you to your local chapter of the National Multiple Sclerosis Society, which can provide a wealth of knowledge and specific resources.)

While each of you will need to examine your own symptoms and employment situation, I encourage you to give yourself some time if you feel uncertain about your ability to continue in your current job. If you have worked long and hard to achieve a current career goal or position, it may be wise to avoid a career-altering decision that is influenced by the initial emotions and challenges of a new diagnosis. The way you feel both physically and mentally will likely be much different (and hopefully improved) six months or one year after your diagnosis. As your symptoms resolve or improve, it is also smart to think about whether making some accommodations would enable you to perform your job more easily. Examples are numerous but include ideas such as:

Can your schedule be adjusted to create some short breaks in your day?
Are there opportunities to work from home one or two days per week?
Would rearrangement of your office space or other work space decrease the
    burden of a new physical problem or symptom?
Is there technology readily available that could assist with particular tasks?
Are there opportunities within your field to work part-time?

Of course, if you decide that you may need some accommodation at work, it is difficult to make this happen without disclosing your diagnosis to your employer. In Chapter 5, I addressed the issues surrounding your decision to tell your employer. If you have decided not to tell your employer but need an adjustment in some aspect of your work, you are going to have to share some pieces of information. You can always refer to a "medical condition" that has caused whatever symptom or disability you have that requires the accommodation. However, speaking in generalizations can get tricky as you try to maintain a sense of trust and honesty with your employer. At that point, your employer may also ask for more information. (Please see more in Chapter 5 on disclosing your diagnosis to coworkers.)

## SHOULD I CONTINUE TO WORK?

Within a few weeks of my diagnosis, it became clear to me that I would be able to continue my job from a physical standpoint. The dizziness was improving and the numbness in my leg was decreasing. Yet, I found myself very worried about whether I *should* work. I certainly enjoyed my job, but I also considered it to be a job that was frequently stressful. Would allowing myself to experience that stress on a daily basis increase my chances of having future relapses? Would keeping up with the busy pace of the emotional and physical challenges of my job every day alter the long-term course of my MS?

The question of whether we *should* work is a very different one to contemplate from that of asking whether we are physically and mentally capable of doing so. While I was not sure in the beginning that I had made the right decision about sticking with my job, seven years later I am sure that it was one of the best things I did for my mental health. As for my physical health, I have not seen any evidence that the daily stress has had any major negative impact on me. However, there are many days when I am more exhausted because I have gone to work that day. In addition, several months ago, I experienced a dramatic increase in fatigue along with an exacerbation of some chronic symptoms. This occurred in the setting of changing to a new job situation and beginning to prepare material for this book. At that time, I was feeling a great deal of stress because of the new responsibilities I had assumed.

That particular exacerbation of chronic symptoms convinced me that stress does have the potential to negatively impact our physical well-being. In fact, a scientific analysis of several studies investigating the effects of stress on multiple sclerosis was reported in the British Medical Journal in 2004.[1] This analysis suggested a correlation between an increase in significant life stressors with an increase in exacerbations for patients with MS. Certainly, this study did not prove cause and effect between stress and MS exacerbations. It does, however, lend support to the notion that excessive stress may take a toll on our health.

If you are concerned about the impact of job stress, consider just how much stress you really experience while at work. A majority of people would probably say that their jobs create some degree of stressful feelings. Do you feel that your stress is excessive? If so, would there be reasonable changes you could make to lessen the stressful environment? In addition, keep in mind that there are many other potential stressors in our lives besides our jobs. While the thought of not working may initially seem like a good way of decreasing overall stress, would it really accomplish this? How would not working impact your financial security? How would it impact your social networks? How would it impact the way you feel about yourself?

Although too much stress on the job may not be in our best health interest, there are clearly tremendous benefits to be derived from continuing to work. Sticking with our career or vocation helps to maintain the sense of self we have developed over the years. Choosing to work provides an opportunity to feel like we are taking some control over a disease whose lack of predictability sometimes makes us worry that we will not always be able to "call the shots." Our jobs give us the opportunity to feel confident that we are still productive members of society. In staying on the job, there is the potential to experience less emotional distress than if we were to choose not to work.

During the past seven years, I have met a great number of wonderful people with relapsing–remitting MS who were diagnosed in the era of disease-modifying drugs. In speaking with them, I have not come across a single person who chose to give up a job solely because of his or her diagnosis. I have definitely spoken with some individuals who made job modifications in order to work around issues of fatigue or disability, or in attempt to decrease stress levels. Of course, this group I refer to is made up of individuals who have had their MS for less than fifteen years and frequently have limited visible disability. This group is also a small sampling of those living with MS based on my own personal encounters. I do suspect that as we track the duration of employment for those of us with MS who started disease-modifying medications at the time of diagnosis, we will see that many of us are able to have longevity in our careers.

## When Real Job Changes Do Need to Be Made

While I do wish to provide a message of encouragement to seek ways to stay with your job, I also realize that the very nature of multiple sclerosis is such that some individuals will not be able to continue performing in their jobs just as they had always done. I personally do not have expertise in the areas of vocational rehabilitation, career or financial counseling, but there is an entire group of people available to you who do. If you anticipate having to make serious changes in your job, or perhaps are contemplating not working at all, I urge you to seek advice from a vocational rehabilitation specialist before you talk to your employer. Once again, your local chapter of the National Multiple

Sclerosis Society will likely be able to assist you in locating such an expert in your area. In addition, the ADA Web site may guide you through some of the background information that will be helpful in understanding the process (www.ada.gov). Keep in mind that the ADA Web site is replete with a great deal of information that may make it somewhat intimidating the first time you navigate your way through it.

If at some point it becomes clear that you will not be able to continue with any line of work, then you will need to become familiar with the process of applying for Social Security Disability Insurance benefits. This is a fairly complex process that is best done under the guidance of someone who has expertise in the area. (More information on this topic is provided in Chapter 12.)

## For Those Who Are Diagnosed before Entering the Workforce

I always take great interest in reading or hearing about the personal stories of others living with MS. As I do so, I have been particularly impressed with students who are diagnosed in their late teens or early twenties when they are still in high school, college, or graduate school. I have read their stories with admiration as they describe persevering through fatigue and various symptoms to see themselves through to graduation. The majority of them seem to anticipate moving forward to their career goals as they had always planned. My random sampling of reading about individuals on Web sites such as "Faces of MS" (www.faceofms.org) does not mean that all students have had such successes. Yet it is clear that there is a sense of determination and hope in many of those who are younger when diagnosed that keeps them moving toward particular goals.

For those who are diagnosed before beginning the journey down a particular career path, the opportunity exists to carefully consider career options. Is a particular job more likely to provide flexibility if and when relapses occur? Is one career more likely to be physically demanding than another? How long are the hours in a typical day with a particular job? While considering these questions is important, I believe the notion of "following your dreams" should not be readily abandoned. There is the possibility of spending the next thirty years or more in a particular line of work. Ideally, your job should be something that you *want* to be doing that can provide personal satisfaction. If I had abandoned my plans to be a physician when I had optic neuritis during my second year of residency training, I think I would look back now and feel that I had cheated myself out of something very important.

## Our Jobs and Who We Are

Our MS is probably going to be with us for a lifetime. We will adjust and adapt to the changes it may or may not bring as our lives unfold. We should be careful not to let the diagnosis stop us from participating in aspects of our lives that reinforce our feelings of self-esteem and self-worth. For those whose careers are already well under way, your job is likely to be one aspect of the way in which you define yourself. For those still considering future jobs, career goals can represent hope for the future. While it may not always be easy as we have to contemplate disclosure on the job and worry about potential discrimination, there is much to be gained from finding the right way to stick with the jobs that have become part of who we are.

# 7

# HAVING CHILDREN

The decision to have children is one of the most intensely personal decisions that a couple or individual will make during a lifetime. Your decision to be a parent incorporates countless different factors, including your own childhood experience, personal values, religious beliefs, career plans, finances, and long-term vision of your life. The diagnosis of multiple sclerosis has the potential to add another layer of complexity to that decision-making process. For some, a life without children cannot be imagined, and there will not be much to contemplate. Others may desire more information as they work their way through what they consider to be a difficult decision. For either group, learning about existing data from the medical community regarding the issues of pregnancy and parenting with MS can provide better understanding and alleviate potential concerns. Admittedly, much of this chapter speaks to women with MS who are contemplating pregnancy. But if you are a man living with MS and considering a future with children, there are sections of this chapter that speak to you as well.

## "SO WHEN WILL YOU HAVE A BABY?"

Approximately three months after my diagnosis, I was attending a family event with my husband and nineteen-month-old daughter. During the visit, a family member made a comment about when my daughter might have a new little brother or sister. While this was an innocent comment without any harmful intentions, I remember feeling so angry. I had just been diagnosed with multiple sclerosis. I was working and had a toddler. Did she not realize that I had enough on my plate at the time? Maybe there would be no more children. It was not that person's business, and I felt angry that she had caused me to think about it.

The truth is that I was still feeling very sorry for myself at that point. I was also in a selfish mindset. I was afraid of making anything worse. While I did not know the specific numbers, I seemed to remember that relapse rates in MS were higher after pregnancy. I felt like it should be *my* decision regarding whether or not I wanted to risk my own health. Not surprisingly, it having been only three months since my diagnosis, I was not willing to begin considering such risks. In addition, my future still seemed so very uncertain. Would I be able physically to take care of children for the next fifteen to twenty years of their lives? I already had one child. Would a second child increase my stress and my chance for relapses over the years?

Six years after those worrisome questions raced through my mind, I live each day with two wonderful daughters. Despite all my fears and concerns, I was able to find satisfactory answers to most of the tough questions I had. Of course, no one held that magic ball to predict the future that we all wish for as we live with MS. Yet, with the information I was able to obtain, my husband and I were able to make a decision about having a second child with much less fear than I had originally experienced.

## WILL PREGNANCY INCREASE MY CHANCES OF HAVING A RELAPSE?

If you are newly diagnosed with MS or have had a recent relapse, the risk of bringing on another exacerbation is likely to be of substantial concern as you contemplate pregnancy. As I gradually began to entertain the possibility of a second child, I found myself quickly retreating to the question of why I would knowingly increase my risk for relapse by having another child. Interestingly, pregnancy itself turns out to be quite favorable in terms of potential relapses. Scientific studies have shown that the number of exacerbations actually decreases during pregnancy, especially after the first trimester.[1] A simple explanation for this phenomenon is that multiple sclerosis is an autoimmune disease, and many different hormones and substances that suppress the immune system are produced by our own bodies during pregnancy.

In contrast to the relative benefits of pregnancy, studies do show an increase in MS exacerbations during the first few months after delivery. The "Pregnancy in Multiple Sclerosis Study" (PRIMS) showed that approximately thirty percent of women experienced a relapse during the first three months postpartum.[1] When I read that report, I immediately felt discouraged and frightened again. However, I decided to go back and read the details of the study because I wondered if the women who had experienced postpartum relapses had gone back on their disease-modifying medications right after delivery. I was surprised to see that none of the women during those first six months postpartum had been on any of the interferon medications or copaxone. Therefore, I wondered if getting back on a disease-modifying medication soon after delivery could prevent the increase in postpartum relapse rates. With that possibility in mind, I again began to feel a little more hopeful about having a second child.

As I delved further into the research on multiple sclerosis and pregnancy, I did come across some encouraging information about the longer-term effects of pregnancy on the course of MS. By the second year postpartum in the PRIMS study, relapse rates were back down to what they had been in the year prior to pregnancy. In addition, follow-up from the PRIMS study suggested that there is no increase in long-term disability in women with MS who choose to have children compared to those who do not.[2]

## DOES HAVING MULTIPLE SCLEROSIS INCREASE MY RISK OF PREGNANCY COMPLICATIONS?

This is a question for which there are many reassuring answers. Having MS does not increase your risk for complications during pregnancy or delivery. MS does not increase the risk for miscarriages, birth defects, preterm delivery, or low-birth-weight children. If you do have a specific disability as a result of your MS prior to becoming pregnant, you will want to weigh the impact of changes in your body during pregnancy on that disability. For example, if you have bladder symptoms prior to pregnancy, there is an excellent chance that these symptoms will intensify with pregnancy, especially during the last trimester. You should also consider any preexisting disability and the potential impact on the delivery process. For example, problems with spasticity in your lower extremities should be discussed with your obstetrician (OB) to ensure a comfortable and smooth delivery. Certainly, the great majority of these issues can be managed with some forethought and planning with your physician.

Should you experience a relapse during pregnancy, most experts seem to agree that intravenous steroids can be used with relative safety. However, this is a decision that would likely be made with your various physicians in consultation with each other (neurologist, obstetrician, and pediatrician) in order to ensure recommendation of what is best for both you and your developing child. Of course, one of the difficult tricks during pregnancy can be trying to determine if a new symptom is coming from MS or is a result of your changing pregnant body.

During my first pregnancy, before I had been diagnosed with MS, I developed sharp shooting pains down my left buttock whenever I walked at a certain pace. This symptom is fairly common during the third trimester of pregnancy when there is additional pressure on the nerve roots in the spinal column. Had I already been diagnosed with MS when I began to experience those electrical shocks, my physician and I may have briefly considered the possibility that I was having a flare of my MS. Fortunately, because I certainly recalled those unpleasant sensations from my first pregnancy, I knew right away that I did not need to worry about an MS exacerbation when those electrical shocks started again during my second pregnancy. (I never promised to paint a glowing picture of all aspects of pregnancy! There will always be challenges during pregnancy that have nothing to do with having MS.)

As I make these efforts to reassure you that multiple sclerosis itself should not have a significant impact on the course of your pregnancy, I must be careful not to generalize too much. The majority of women with MS who are making decisions about having children are relatively young and are unlikely to have accumulated significant disabilities. However, if you are someone who already has a challenging disability, then your pregnancy may have some different issues related to your specific disability. This, of course, does not mean that you should never become pregnant. It just means that a preconception consultation with an obstetrician should be considered in order to allow for appropriate planning of pregnancy needs.

## WHAT ARE THE CHANCES OF PASSING MULTIPLE SCLEROSIS ALONG TO MY CHILD?

As I moved past my selfish concerns about having a second child, the extremely burdensome worry about the potential to pass this illness along to my children resurfaced. By then, many tears had already been shed as I considered the possibility that my first little girl would have an increased risk of MS because of me. As soon as your children are born, you begin to have many hopes and dreams for their futures. More than anything, you want happiness for your child. The idea of passing along any type of illness to one's children can create some powerful feelings of guilt as well as excessive worry for their well-being.

I again decided to get the facts about how likely I would be to pass the illness along to my children. "The facts" in this area are not as crystal clear as we might want them to be, but there are still some well-calculated numbers to consider. As a very general rule, the risk of anyone developing multiple sclerosis is approximately 1 in every 750 people. The risk for a child whose parent has MS is about 1 in 40. Keep in mind, if multiple family members have had MS, then the chances for a child in that family may be higher than 1 in 40. While some genes have been identified that are more common in people with MS, there has yet to be a single gene identified that is solely responsible for MS. Current thinking is that an individual may be born with a genetic predisposition for MS that is then "turned on" by some environmental factors that have yet to be determined.

I must say that I felt absolutely no comfort in coming upon the above statistics. While a 1-in-40 chance of developing an illness did not sound terrible, it sounded much worse than 1 in 750. The numbers sound particularly bothersome when you are the one responsible for changing those odds for your own child. As I began to feel ready to have a second child for many other wonderful reasons, I spent a lot of time rationalizing those numbers. Yes, my children will have an increased risk of MS compared to the general population. But, think how far MS research will have come by the time they are in their twenties or thirties. Certainly, we should be very good at controlling the disease by then. Perhaps, we will even have a cure. I also convinced myself that a 1-in-40 chance was still pretty good odds. Lastly, I knew without any reservation that

I would rather be living on this planet with MS than not be here at all. I would hope that my children would feel the same way.

If you do have several family members with MS, a consultation with a genetic counselor may be very helpful. A counselor may be able to provide additional guidance regarding risk for MS in your children. Currently, testing for genetic susceptibility to MS is not being done, but that may change in the near future. However, a genetic counselor would look for any inheritance patterns in your own family and apply what we currently know about the genetics of MS to your particular situation.

## WILL I BE ABLE TO ADEQUATELY CARE FOR MY CHILDREN?

This is where it would be particularly helpful to have that magic crystal ball to predict our future. If we could be sure that our level of disability would be minimal over the next fifteen years, our worries about being able to take care of our children would obviously be much less. For those with a spouse or significant other in your life, it is crucial to have an open discussion with that person regarding what his or her role in child rearing will be. Even in the absence of MS, it is very helpful for couples to plan ahead regarding who will be doing the child care and how that will fit into your work and home lifestyles. When one partner does have MS and you discuss the "what ifs" down the road, it is important for the partner without MS to understand that he or she may have to take on greater child care responsibilities at some point if your health status were to change.

While these conversations are important to have with your partner, I personally believe that you can never anticipate and plan for every future event in your life, whether you live with MS or not. The majority of couples choosing to have children know that there are never any guarantees for the health or welfare of either parent. Once I had been diagnosed with MS, my husband and I knew that we could not predict what the future held for my health. Yet, we knew that we were committed to each other and any children we might have. We would tackle the various "bumps in the road" as they emerged over time.

If you are already living with disability from your MS, then some additional planning for the specific challenges you may face with a new baby will likely be needed. If you are uncertain where to turn for such assistance, an occupational therapist may be a good place to start for evaluation of your specific needs as you care for an infant. Of course, the infant stage is only one of many stages. Future, first-time parents tend to focus primarily on the baby that will be arriving. However, as you anticipate some of your own needs, keep in mind that your child is going to pass through many different stages during the first five years of his life. He will transform from a highly dependent infant with many physical needs to a physically independent five-year-old with many emotional needs. Therefore, a particular disability may not always have the same implications for your ability to care for your child as he grows and changes.

## Children, Stress, and Fatigue

Even without an existing physical disability, there is little doubt that having a child will add to your level of fatigue. All new parents are fatigued during the first few months of their baby's life, whether they have a chronic illness or not. It is truly amazing how a little tiny person can completely turn your entire schedule upside down and inside out. Yet, even as children grow and sleep through the night, there are physically tiring aspects of raising children that persist for many years. There are baths to be given, strollers to be lifted in and out of cars, games of tag to be played, and countless other highly enjoyable but potentially exhausting activities to be done.

Contemplating the ability to keep up with the busy lives of children may begin to sound quite stressful. I would be dishonest if I were to say that my children were never a source of stress for me. Of course they are. I love them tremendously, and I want what is best for them. I want them to feel that they are getting what they need from me. Yet in the day-to-day reality of living with my girls, there is a lot of giving to be done. I do not always feel up to the task of giving of myself every minute of every day. I realize that all parents feel this way with some regularity. Nonetheless, I do believe that there are days when the symptoms of my MS make the giving of myself to my children that much more difficult.

While it may be good to have a sense of "what you are in for" as you contemplate having children, there is another *incredibly important* side of the story to be told about having children. For all the giving that is done for your children, the receiving side can never be adequately described. There are few greater joys in life than to have an infant cuddled up on your shoulder, to be smothered in kisses by your adoring three-year-old or to take part in the endless giggles of a silly situation. While I know that my stress levels certainly go up because of my children, it is also my children who bring those levels down better than anyone else. Although I will never be able to prove it, I suspect that having my children in my life is far better for my health than if I were not to have them.

## Practical Considerations for Pregnancy

### Should I Take My MS Medications While Trying to Become Pregnant?

Once my husband and I decided that we were going to have another child, I began to worry about coming off my medication for the duration of time that I would be trying to become pregnant. I knew that it had taken about six months to become pregnant with my first child. I worried about potential relapses if

I were off medication and it took that long to conceive again. The recommendations from the pharmaceutical manufacturers of the disease-modifying MS drugs state that the three interferon medications (Avonex, Betaseron, and Rebif) as well as Copaxone should not be taken while pregnant or while trying to become pregnant. Because of these recommendations, it is best to speak with your neurologist once you know you are planning to become pregnant. Having him involved in the discussion about when to come off medication will be helpful in your own decision-making process. Your neurologist may even have some thoughts on the timing of your pregnancy based on the recent activity of your MS. Current recommendations state that men with MS may stay on their disease-modifying medication while their significant other is trying to conceive.

My personal approach to taking disease-modifying medication while trying to conceive is not one that I can safely recommend to women since it is not consistent with formal recommendations. However, I choose to share the details of what I did because I know that there are some women who will struggle with medication decisions during the period of time that they are trying to become pregnant. Because I was very reluctant to stop my disease-modifying medication for what could turn out to be six months or more, I decided that I would begin very careful record keeping of each monthly menstrual cycle. I purchased ovulation kits so that I could increase the likelihood of becoming pregnant. With each cycle, I took my injection medication from the first day of my period until I had ovulated that month. Once I had tried to conceive for that month, I did not restart my medication until another menstrual cycle began.

Essentially, I was taking my medication for a little more than half of each month. I had absolutely no scientific data on which to base this. There were no studies to tell me how effective my medication was when I was only taking it fifty percent of the time. There were also no studies to tell me that this would be safe for a future child. However, in taking this somewhat unconventional approach, I maintained a sense of control in continuing to treat my MS. Importantly, it also removed some of the pressure in terms of feeling the need to become pregnant immediately since I was still partially taking my medication.

Again, I do not share my approach so that everyone will descend upon their neurologists with this plan in mind. What is important is to realize is that each individual will have different levels of comfort in choosing when to come off medications during that period of time prior to becoming pregnant. An open discussion with your neurologist and obstetrician will enable you to come up with a plan that feels most comfortable for you.

Recommendations are clear that women should remain off the disease-modifying drugs for the duration of their pregnancy. Because relapse rates decrease during pregnancy, you may feel less concerned about being off medications during the pregnancy itself. Once I was pregnant with my second child, I became very focused on growing a healthy child. For all my prepregnancy concerns about relapse, I hardly gave it any thought during those nine months. And I must admit, I definitely enjoyed taking a break from the injections.

### When Should I Restart My Medications after I Deliver?

The answer to this question depends on whether or not you are planning to breastfeed. It is not clear how much of the disease-modifying drugs enter breast milk, and current recommendations are not to take them while breast-feeding. From the standpoint of your child's health, breast milk is clearly the best nutrition you can provide during those early months. However, it also important for the well-being of a child to have a healthy mother. The question therefore becomes whether you remain off disease-modifying medication during the first few months postpartum when relapse rates are known to increase in order to provide optimal nutrition for your child.

Many women have very strong feelings about breastfeeding, independent of the potential issue of taking medication while nursing. If you have always believed that breastfeeding is the best way to go, then staying off medication will be an easier choice for you to make. I struggled quite a bit with the best course of action to take since my preference was for my daughter to have the nutrition of breast milk. Unfortunately, I had a very difficult time breastfeeding my first child and was only able to nurse for three to four months. While I very much wanted my second child to receive every bit of nutrition that her big sister had, I also knew that breastfeeding had not been easy for me. Ultimately, I decided to breastfeed my second child for one month so that she would receive many of the good antibodies that come with the earlier milk. I then planned to get back on my medication as soon as I stopped breastfeeding. Of course, I had a much easier time breastfeeding my second child, but I stuck with my one-month plan nonetheless!

Currently, we do not have any clear-cut answers to give women as to what they should do about timing for reinitiation of disease-modifying medication versus duration of breastfeeding. Women in the PRIMS study who breastfed their children did not have a higher rate of relapse than women who did not. You should gather the opinions of both your neurologist and your future pediatrician and weigh them in the context of your own feelings. If you place a very high priority on breastfeeding, you should not feel compelled to abandon it. Choosing to breastfeed and to stay off medications certainly does not guarantee a relapse. On the other hand, if you choose not to breastfeed, getting back on medications after delivery would be a sensible option.

## THE JOY OF CHILDREN

While you and your partner ponder the statistics and consider how children might fit into your lives, I feel compelled to share a few personal thoughts on what having children has meant for me. When I first got married, I had absolutely no maternal instinct. I would see children begging for candy in the check-out lanes at the grocery store or throwing tantrums in the middle of the mall. I could not imagine why happy couples would choose to bring that craziness into their lives. Then, after five years of marriage and the realization that we were not getting any younger, my husband and I began to feel that children were in fact part of our long-term vision.

Now, as a mother of two daughters, I cannot imagine life without them. I love them more than I ever thought possible. While every day has many challenging moments because of them, every single day also has great joy because of them. They have taught me many things about myself as I figure out how to help them. They keep my mind active with their incredibly perceptive questions, and they keep my body active as I kick a soccer ball with them or teach them how to ride a two-wheeler.

As I said at the beginning of this chapter, the decision to have children is intensely personal. While children have become a very important part of my own life, I could not possibly predict what is right for someone else's life. My goal in writing this chapter was to answer many of the questions that emerge as you factor the role of multiple sclerosis in to that very important and personal decision.

# 8

# Staying Healthy and Fit

Depending on where you are in finding a comfort level with your diagnosis of MS, you may be ready to think about ways you can maintain your health through diet, exercise, and other alternative therapies. Some of you may be very eager to learn answers to common questions when facing a new diagnosis: "Are there particular foods I can eat to stay healthier? What exercises can I do? Are there vitamins or supplements that are effective in helping to control MS?" Others may feel that you have already had enough challenges with injection medications, possible side effects, and lifestyle changes that you are not ready to modify the comfortable aspects of your routine such as the foods you eat.

A simple answer for both groups of people is that there are no definite, scientifically proven foods, exercise programs or supplements that will dramatically alter the course of your MS. However, I firmly believe that if we do what we can to keep ourselves healthy and strong, any future relapses will be less of a burden to a body that is otherwise in good physical condition. I am fairly certain that the heat-induced weakness I sometimes experience in my leg might really cause my leg to drag if those muscles were not kept in reasonable shape. And YES, there is some scientific evidence that certain exercises and dietary changes can make small but important improvements for those living with multiple sclerosis.

I am certainly not suggesting that we all get personal trainers, which would be great if you were that motivated or this were an affordable option, or start dieting to look like super models, which would not be healthy at all! What I am suggesting is that some form of exercise become a regular part of your weekly routine. In combination with exercise, learning to make healthy food choices every day can lead to a body that is truly in better physical condition. Keep in mind that just because we have MS, this does not mean that other diseases cannot come our way in the future. While we had no control in preventing the onset of our MS, we do have the ability to prevent or delay certain illnesses like diabetes and high blood pressure by maintaining healthy lifestyles.

Sounding like a doctor preaching to patients is never my intention in this book. I am on *your* side with this. Every day, I realize how much easier it is to talk about healthy eating and getting regular exercise than it is to actually do it. I am definitely not the ideal role model for healthy habits all the time. There are times of the year when several weeks can slip by and I realize I have not exercised at all. There are nights when we take our kids out for ice cream that I simply cannot pass up a hot fudge sundae. Yet, I do know that I feel better physically and mentally during those periods of time that I am exercising and eating well—my mind seems a little sharper, my fatigue is truly decreased, and my outlook seems brighter.

## EXERCISE

### Too Tired to Exercise

For those of us living with multiple sclerosis, fatigue is a common symptom. At times, this fatigue can even feel disabling. So how are we supposed to exercise when walking itself feels burdensome on certain days? And, aren't we supposed to avoid getting overheated? Is it really okay to exercise, and can it really be helpful? Interestingly, some scientific studies have been done to try to answer some of these important questions.

One study compared people with MS who were participating either in a yoga or an aerobic exercise program (on a stationary bike) versus people who did not participate in any regular exercise. After six months of participation, those doing either yoga or aerobic exercise reported *less* fatigue when compared to those who were not doing any exercise program.[1] While it may be counterintuitive at first, it does seem that if we can just get ourselves started in some sort of exercise routine, we may actually have decreased levels of fatigue in the long run. Not surprisingly, other studies have shown that people with MS with mild to moderate disability can improve their walking speed and upper and lower body strength with a regular aerobic exercise program.[2]

The idea of exercising to potentially decrease fatigue is a hard concept to put into practice. If you are going to have any success at all, it is critical to find an exercise program that really works for you as an individual.

### Finding the Right Exercise for You

Regardless of whether or not you experience significant fatigue with your MS, finding time for regular exercise is a challenge for everyone. Therefore, your exercise program truly needs to have a good personal fit. It has to be a type of exercise that works best for your schedule, your level of fatigue, and your current physical abilities. Consider the following questions as you contemplate a potential exercise routine.

### *What Kinds of Exercise Might I Actually Enjoy Doing?*

First and foremost, you have to *like* the type of exercise you choose. For many years, even before I had MS, I would run to stay fit. Yet the reality is that I hated running. I always dreaded going out to exercise. Not enjoying the type of exercise you choose is obviously going to decrease your level of enthusiasm for the process.

As you think about the many options for exercise, consider what appeals to you as well as what might fit best with your current physical abilities. Are you a walker, runner, biker, or swimmer? Do you prefer to exercise in a class setting with an instructor? Do you like working out on specific types of equipment such as treadmills, elliptical machines, or stair climbers? Or, perhaps it is finally time to give yoga a try now that you know there can truly be some benefits.

Several years ago, I met another physician with MS who became frustrated with the fact that he could not run well anymore after years of competitive running. For a period of time, he did not exercise at all. Interestingly, during that time he also stopped taking his MS medications. He did not recognize that he had become depressed and was ignoring all aspects of his health. A relatively minor relapse of his MS came as a wake up call to him. He got back on his medications and began to ride a bike instead of running. Of course this benefited his physical health, but he said the change in his mental health was even better. Regular exercise seemed to provide him with an emotional lift.

If you find yourself wondering what type of exercise you can do because of a new disability, there are countless resources to assist you. Most neighborhood fitness centers have trainers who can help to provide ideas and options. Sometimes, a consultation with a physical therapist or someone at a rehabilitation facility can be of great benefit. A trained therapist can help to tailor an exercise program to your likes and abilities. I also refer you to the National Multiple Sclerosis Society's brochure on exercise, which has a section on specific options for those living with MS. It is so important not to let a mild to moderate physical disability become a bigger disability, both physically and mentally, by deciding that you cannot exercise.

### *When Will I Exercise?*

Especially for those who have a significant degree of fatigue, this is another important question to consider as you plan an exercise routine. Most of us have times of day when our energy level seems to be better and we are more likely to be successful in getting ourselves to exercise. There is no way I could ever consider exercising at the end of a workday. I am physically exhausted. I do better midmornings on days when I do not go to work. In addition to thinking about a time of day when your energy level might be best, there will always be the practical considerations about when to exercise that have to do with your own personal schedule. Unfortunately, that window of time when your personal schedule opens up may not always correspond with your best energy times. Try not to let that be a reason for not exercising at all. Some exercise is always better than none.

### How Often Should I Exercise and for How Long?

My personal feeling on this is that you should never feel like you have to live up to certain prespecified targets in terms of number of minutes exercised each session or total days of the week exercised. What I have found to be so amazing about living with MS is that I really do have a different body on different days and during different months. There are days that even with the best of intentions, I feel like I am really dragging after fifteen minutes of exercise. Other days, I will be out walking with a friend and I am still going strong thirty minutes into a brisk walk. Above all, *listen to your body.*

If exercise is new to you altogether, starting slowly is important. Even if you have been a serious athlete throughout your life, give yourself a break if you are just getting back into a routine after some time off with a new diagnosis. If ten minutes is all you do each session for the first few weeks, that is more than you were doing before. Every one to two weeks, you can slowly increase the amount of time you spend exercising. At some point, your body is likely to tell you what duration of time works best for you. Whenever I choose to exercise on the elliptical machine, it takes about twenty minutes until my right leg starts to become numb and feel like a dead weight. So even though I know I could continue to push my cardiovascular system past those twenty minutes, I never do because I am trying to listen to all parts of my body.

While daily exercise is ideal, it simply is not realistic for everyone. I encourage everyone to begin by looking for three days each week to exercise. If you have not exercised in a long time, three days per week is a great start. If you are able to stick with it and start to notice the benefits of exercise, there is a chance you will find time on other days to slip in a few minutes of exercise. However, as I said earlier, in living with MS, the same body does not always show up to exercise each time. If you are not having one of your better days, then give yourself a break and try again the next day.

### Making Exercise Fun

Having fun while exercising can have everything to do with the success of your personal program. While the most important part of making exercise fun may be in choosing the right type of exercise for yourself, there are a few other ways to keep it fun. For me, music makes all the difference. I have a number of motivating, high-energy songs that I listen to whenever I exercise alone. The music helps my feet to keep moving and passes the time quickly. I cannot imagine getting through twenty minutes on the elliptical machine without it.

Another way to make exercise fun is to turn it into a social event. I have a friend that I walk with whenever we can get our schedules to line up. We always have so much news to catch up on that the time passes quickly and I forget that I am exercising. Before my schedule became so hectic, I used to love going to group exercise classes. The fellowship of working hard at something with a group of peers provided a lot of great satisfaction.

If a group class sounds like fun to you, but you are worried about having to take a break if a symptom starts to bother you, strongly consider telling the instructor about your MS. I was in an adult figure skating class five years ago, but could never do the spins because I have lost the ability to maintain my balance if I spin. I decided to tell the instructor about my situation. Because I did not know the other women in the class very well, I just told them I had a medical problem that prevented me from spinning. Fortunately, because we are adults, others are very unlikely to ask questions or to be critical if we modify our activities in a group class.

## Keeping Cool, Literally

For the first few years that I had MS, I would hear others talk about their symptoms getting worse in the heat, but I had never experienced it myself. However, as I began to exercise more regularly, and after a few summers of living in North Carolina, I began to notice that my arm and leg numbness really did amplify whenever I let myself get overheated. Worsening of chronic or intermittent symptoms in the heat is a well-known phenomenon with MS. Nerve fibers that have lost myelin do not conduct as well when our core body temperature rises. Increased weakness, fatigue, numbness, or exacerbation of other symptoms really can occur in an overheated body.

Because of this heat-induced phenomenon, keeping cool as best as we can is very important when we exercise. While we cannot exercise without some elevation of our core body temperature, there are many strategies to keep the heat away. Choose air-conditioned facilities during the warmer months of the year and save outside activities for the cooler months of the year or cooler times of day. Many fitness centers have large overhead fans or floor fans throughout the gym. I try to exercise on equipment near a fan whenever possible. Dressing in layers also helps so that you can remove a layer as you feel your body heating up. Keeping cold water on hand and taking mini-breaks for a very cold drink when you start to heat up will also help.

When it comes to getting overheated with exercise, once again, *listen to your body.* There is no point in pushing yourself to finish forty-five minutes on the stationary bike if your leg is going to drag behind the rest of your body as you walk off the bike. In living with MS, the right amount of exercise can have definite physical and mental benefits. Pushing yourself to excess heat and exhaustion will not.

The good news is that if we do unintentionally find ourselves with exacerbation of symptoms in the setting of getting overheated from exercise, these symptoms usually do not last more than several minutes to a few hours. Cooling down after exercise, whether you have experienced heat-related symptoms or not, is very important too. Look for a cool room, fan, pool, or shower (not hot) after you exercise. Continue to drink cold water as you cool down. Your feet and head also hold a lot of heat. So take off any shoes, socks, or caps you may be wearing as you cool down your body.

## CHOOSING HEALTHY FOODS

I specifically chose not to use the subheading "Diet" for this section. *Diet* is a word in our society that makes us think that we will be restricted in what we eat, or that we will be eating foods that we really would rather not be eating. If we search for solid scientific evidence about what to eat or not to eat with multiple sclerosis, there is no specific "MS diet" that is going to prevent relapses or improve existing symptoms. So if you really love ice cream or some other food, no one is going to suggest that you give it up altogether.

However, just as with exercise, while there may not be a specific diet we can follow to improve the health of our nervous system, choosing foods that allow us to maintain a healthy weight and good cardiovascular health will likely help us in the long run. Just as I truly believe that a physically fit body will better tolerate and compensate for any future relapses, a body that is at a healthy weight should also fare better. Imagine the additional burden of trying to walk with a 250-pound body instead of a 150-pound body if suddenly one of your legs were to become weak.

### How Do I Know What a Healthy Weight Is for Me?

My example of the two weights above may not be appropriate if you happen to be six feet tall. Of course, it would not be healthy for someone six feet tall to weigh only 150 pounds. One of the best ways you can determine a good weight range for yourself is to learn about your current body mass index (BMI). Depending on your bone structure, a person's BMI should run in the range of 19–24 kg/m$^2$. While there is a formula that calculates BMI, you can readily look up your BMI on a chart by using your height and weight. Most primary care physician offices have BMI charts readily available, or you can quickly determine your BMI by searching "body mass index calculator" on the internet.

### What Do You Mean by "Healthy Eating"?

If you try to keep up with the volumes of information that appear each year on what constitutes healthy eating and what does not, you may sometimes feel overwhelmed. For a long time, we were told that low-fat diets were the healthiest. Then, we learned that there were "good fats" and "bad fats." This was followed by a highly publicized shift toward decreasing our carbohydrates and replacing white carbohydrates with healthier, brown, whole-grain carbohydrates.

Certain aspects of all of the above may be true. There are excellent nutritional advisory resources that can help to clarify all of the mixed messages we receive. The U.S. Department of Agriculture's food pyramid provides an excellent guide to healthy eating. Their Web site can even assist you in developing a personalized eating plan (www.mypyramid.gov). The National MS Society also has a comprehensive brochure with detailed information on what constitutes healthy eating. A one-on-one consultation with a registered dietician is another option that can result in a personalized eating plan that works best for your lifestyle. Depending on your insurance plan, a visit with a dietician may be a covered benefit.

### Using Food for Comfort

Good food can truly be a source of comfort for some of us when we are under emotional stress. Others will eat less during stress. If you are one of those who chooses food as a means of stress relief, it is very important not to allow the stress of a new diagnosis of MS promote comfort eating habits indefinitely. During the first few months after my diagnosis, maintaining a healthy weight was the farthest thing from my mind. I do not think I was consciously choosing to eat more. I just knew that I was not going to deprive myself of any food that I really wanted since life was otherwise not seeming so kind at the time.

In the long run though, I have tried to use MS as one of my main motivational factors for eating well and maintaining an appropriate weight. Maintaining my weight allows me to worry a little less about issues such a possible diabetes or high blood pressure. And even though I cannot prove it, I like to believe that a healthy weight will be better for the course of my MS over the years.

## VITAMINS, SUPPLEMENTS, AND OTHER NATURAL REMEDIES

### What Vitamins Can I Take that Would Be Beneficial for Multiple Sclerosis? Are There Specific Supplements I Should Consider Taking?

During the past ten to fifteen years, the field of complementary and alternative medicine has taken off in our country. As consumers, we have been very interested in learning all we can about what vitamins and supplements might help us live longer and healthier lives. So it is not surprising that when many of us are diagnosed with multiple sclerosis, we are very interested in learning about what types of "natural" supplements might be good for us. I think this is particularly true because most of us are learning how to do a self-injection medication. We maintain that little bit of hope that perhaps some "nontraditional" medication or supplement might be able to do an adequate job of controlling our MS and spare us from the injection therapy. Even though I intended to do my injection medication, I spent many hours on my computer during the first few months of my diagnosis, researching all the different types of supplement options.

While I promise to share my thoughts on a few specific supplements, I must first provide a *message of caution.* Please remember that any supplement, vitamin, or other "natural" food product that is not in the form of a prescription from a doctor does not come with the same extensive safety and efficacy evaluation as a prescription drug that has been approved by the Food and Drug Administration (FDA). Fortunately, many vitamins and supplements are now being evaluated in scientific studies. However, as a consumer, it may be very hard to know which supplements have been carefully investigated. Therefore, I strongly recommend the following before you begin a supplement or any natural product:

1. Talk to your neurologist about the supplement. There is an excellent chance that he may be aware of risks and benefits based on recent scientific studies. Your neurologist may also have had the opportunity to see how other patients have responded to the supplement you are considering. (I think many patients are afraid to ask their doctors about "alternative" therapies. You may worry that your doctor will think you are not taking his recommendations seriously. Or, you may worry that he will think you are foolish for pursuing nontraditional therapies. I can assure you that in the current era of medicine, doctors have become very accustomed to their patients' asking about alternative therapies. With MS in particular, it is quite common for patients to ask these questions. Your neurologist may have an opinion to help guide you in your decision on whether or not to take the supplement.)

2. Educate yourself about the supplement. I have found the Rocky Mountain MS Center Web site to be very comprehensive and fair in evaluating hundreds of complementary and alternative therapies for MS: www.ms-cam.org. The authors for this Web site also frequently write articles about complementary therapies in the National Multiple Sclerosis Society magazine called, "Inside MS."

3. Be careful of *immune-boosting* supplements. Remember that MS is an autoimmune disease—our own immune systems are attacking the myelin coating our nerve fibers. So taking herbs or vitamins to turn up our immune systems has the potential to be harmful. No study has ever proven this to be the case. Nevertheless, without a good reason to take them, it may be best to avoid them.

4. Avoid fraud. Just as there are countless makers of the latest and greatest supplement to help you lose weight as you see advertised on the flyers inside the weekend newspaper, there are also people out there trying to get rich by taking advantage of patients with various illnesses. Be wary of those charging large sums of money for supplements or treatments sold right out of their own office. Look into the credentials of the person selling the supplements. Ask for names of those who have already taken the supplements. If someone is unwilling to provide references, then I would not be comfortable with that situation.

### *Vitamin D and Calcium*

Vitamin D has received a lot of attention regarding its potential role in multiple sclerosis. One scientific study reported in 2006 suggested that Caucasians with high levels of vitamin D had a lower risk of developing MS.[3] Experiments have also shown that a disease similar to MS in mice can be prevented with high levels of vitamin D.[4] However, for those of us who already have multiple sclerosis the important question is whether vitamin D can still be of any help to us now.

I believe there are several good reasons to consider taking a vitamin D supplement if you have MS. The most important reason is indirectly related to MS and actually has to do with our bones. Both calcium and vitamin D are critical for maintenance of our bone strength over the years. Particularly for women living with MS, we will experience an increased rate of bone loss as we go through our menopausal years and beyond. However, waiting until our bones are already thinning as we go through menopause is probably not the smartest approach to take. Trying to maintain bone strength in our premenopausal years is a better preventive measure.

Strong bones are just as important to have as strong muscles for the overall fitness of your body in living with MS. Some of us with MS may develop changes in the way we walk over the years that can create an increased risk for falling. Even though the way I walk is normal most of the time, I find myself tripping over my right foot one or two times every week. If one of those trips ever leads to an actual fall, I want my bones to be as strong as possible so I do not find myself with a broken wrist or hip.

Surprisingly, there are thousands of men and women in our country who are unknowingly deficient in vitamin D. While many foods are fortified with vitamin D, sunlight remains our greatest source of vitamin D. Therefore, those living in cooler climates at higher latitudes are at increased risk for vitamin D deficiency. There is also an association between growing up in a part of the country at a higher latitude and developing multiples sclerosis. Many now believe that at least part of the reason for this association is the lower levels of vitamin D in those living at higher latitudes.

Beyond increasing our bone strength, there is not yet any strong scientific evidence that vitamin D supplements can decrease relapse rates or future disability for those of us already living with MS. However, because vitamin D appears to play a role in MS onset, and because we all need to maximize our bone strength, taking calcium with vitamin D should be strongly considered. Under age fifty, 1000 mg of calcium per day is recommended and can be obtained through both diet and supplements. Over age fifty, 1200–1500 mg of calcium per day is needed. Vitamin D (400–800 IU/day) can be taken as an individual supplement, in combination with a calcium supplement pill or as part of a daily multivitamin.

### Omega-3 Fatty Acids

During the current time in which I am writing this book, the "omega-3's" are getting a lot of press because of their ability to lower cholesterol and their potential benefit in multiple sclerosis. I chose to include a small section on them because the omega-3 fatty acids *may* have potential health benefits whether you have MS or not.

What on earth are the "omega-3's?" They are one type of polyunsaturated fat. These days, we talk about the good fats and the bad fats, another one of those confusing pieces of information about healthy eating. The polyunsaturated fatty acids are the good fats and are sometimes called "PUFAs" for short. Both omega-3 and omega-6 are polyunsaturated fats that our bodies do not make so we need to get them in our diet in foods such as fatty fish (like salmon), flaxseed, and canola oil. Because it is hard to get a reasonable amount of these in your diet every day, some people choose to take fish oil supplements.

Since omega-3 fatty acids play a role in the functioning of the immune system, a few scientific studies have looked at patients with relapsing–remitting MS to see if taking fish oil supplements might prevent relapses. While the results of these studies suggested that fewer relapses occurred in those taking fish oil, the studies were conducted in such a way that conclusions about fish oil being the main factor in the decreased number of relapses could not be certain.[5,6]

Because we have limited information about the benefits of the omega-3 fatty acids thus far, you should definitely talk to your neurologist if you are thinking about taking fish oil supplements. She may feel there is enough potential for benefit to make it worth your while. If you happen to have high cholesterol, you may have another reason to consider the supplement since they may also help to balance your good and bad cholesterol. The omega-3 fatty acids can thin the blood slightly, so your primary care physician should also know if you choose to take them.

## An Opportunity

While doing our part to stay healthy and fit can be a challenge, I think we need to view this as another opportunity to positively impact the course of our MS. While I have not identified any specific diet or exercise program that will prevent future relapses, I suspect that our long-term disability may be slightly less if we keep ourselves physically fit. I realize that it can be hard to exercise *today* with the hope that your ability to walk will be better *ten years* from now. Yet, the payoffs truly can be appreciated in the present. As most aspects of learning to live with MS take time, be patient with yourself in finding the exercise program that feels good to you and makes you feel good about yourself.

*Whenever I come to the end of a brisk thirty-minute walk, my right leg always feels prickly and heavy. My heart pounds in my chest, and I am aware of the air rushing in and out of my lungs. I am very much alive. I feel good.*

# 9

# MANAGING THE FATIGUE
# OF MULTIPLE SCLEROSIS

Fatigue—one of the most troubling but invisible symptoms of multiple sclerosis. It has been reported, depending on the source, that between 65 and 95 percent of people living with MS report fatigue as one of their symptoms. Even more problematic is that 15 to 40 percent of people describe it as the most disabling of their symptoms. Just what is this fatigue of multiple sclerosis, why do we have it, and what can we do about it?

Figuring out why we experience fatigue in MS has been a complex issue for the doctors and researchers to resolve. While it is very easy to measure something like how long it takes us to walk twenty yards, it is extremely difficult to measure or study the level of fatigue that we feel. As patients, it may also be difficult for us to find the right words to accurately describe the overwhelming fatigue that some of us experience.

To further complicate the issue of fatigue, physicians may sometimes refer to two kinds of fatigue in MS. *Primary fatigue* is fatigue that cannot be explained by any other cause besides the underlying MS. *Secondary fatigue* can be explained by some other process such as sleeping problems, heat exposure, medication adverse effects, or depression. Because an individual may have a component of primary fatigue that is worsened by a secondary cause, it is important to speak with your doctor in attempting to work through the various possibilities in your particular case.

Although I cited a high percentage of people with MS who experience fatigue, keep in mind that not everyone with MS experiences fatigue. If you are reading this and thinking that you really do not have much fatigue, please don't feel like you should suddenly start experiencing it! Perhaps having been very fit and in the habit of regular exercise prior to a diagnosis is beneficial in terms of having less fatigue with MS. More likely, the varying symptoms of multiple sclerosis in different individuals accounts for the variability seen in levels of fatigue. If you have not experienced much fatigue to date, maintaining healthy dietary, exercise, and sleep habits are the logical steps in keeping fatigue at bay.

## PRIMARY FATIGUE IN MULTIPLE SCLEROSIS

Three years ago, I was asked to speak about fatigue in multiple sclerosis to a small group of individuals living with MS. At that time, fatigue was a part of my everyday experience and was negatively impacting my quality of life. I described my fatigue to them as follows:

> On most days around 1:00 P.M., a very heavy cloud of fatigue starts to take over. This is not the type of tired that allows me to yawn and keep going. This is not the kind of tired that I used to feel at the end of a busy day. This feels like a weight pulling my whole body down. I feel as though I have been drugged and will have to go to sleep in order to recover. This is the kind of fatigue that on many days makes me wonder how I am going to make it until 3:00 P.M.

The fatigue of multiple sclerosis has been described as total body exhaustion. It can be a lack of physical energy, mental energy, or both. Sometimes, there may be a sense of total inability to continue with a particular task, more because of fatigue than because of other physical symptoms from MS. Interestingly, the level of fatigue can be out of proportion to a person's level of disability. One might think that an individual exerting great physical effort to walk with a cane or a walker would be more fatigued than someone who has minimal physical disability. Yet, the fatigue of MS can be just as problematic for the person who has minor or no physical disability.

Enduring this kind of fatigue on a regular basis could certainly create a sense of hopelessness if it were never treated. You may have noticed that I described my experience with severe fatigue as something that occurred in the past. Due to a number of different interventions during the past few years, I no longer encounter severe fatigue on a daily basis. I am not completely free of fatigue, but I am greatly improved from three years ago. By carefully examining your situation for other possible factors contributing to your fatigue, and by making subsequent lifestyle adjustments, you can appreciably decrease the fatigue you experience. However, because many individuals still have significant "primary fatigue" after all the potential secondary causes have been treated, it is important to know that there are prescription medications available to help with this fatigue as well.

## WHAT CAUSES PRIMARY FATIGUE IN MS?

There are many theories as to why the disease process of multiple sclerosis itself may cause fatigue. Some of these theories have to do with increased levels of inflammatory proteins called cytokines in patients with MS. Cytokines may induce feelings of fatigue. Other theories attribute fatigue to loss of the nerve fibers called axons that send signals within the brain. Currently, these ideas are still under investigation and no one can say with certainty what causes the fatigue.

## LOOKING FOR SECONDARY CAUSES OF FATIGUE

Because there is the potential for taking a number of different prescription medications over time as we live with MS, I am a strong proponent of looking for other possible causes of fatigue before beginning a medication to combat it. Usually, there is not just one single reason that someone experiences fatigue in living with MS. Most of the time, there will be a few different reasons. I encourage you to review the list of questions below. Look for changes you can readily make on your own. Other solutions are going to require assistance from your physician.

### Is Poor Sleep Contributing to Fatigue?

The very first question I ask any patient who is experiencing fatigue, whether they have MS or not, is whether they feel they are "getting a good night's sleep." We cannot expect to have normal levels of energy during the day if we are not sleeping well at night. There are so many different types of sleep disorders that there is now a distinct medical specialty called "Sleep Medicine." Some of these sleep disorders may be related to having MS, while many of them are common in the general population.

You can carefully examine your sleep habits and determine if there are areas for possible intervention by review of the following questions:

Do you have trouble falling asleep at night?
Do you wake up in the middle of the night and have trouble falling back to sleep?
If you do wake up in the middle of the night, is there something specific such as the need to use the bathroom that causes you to wake?
If you have a bed partner, does he or she report that you snore excessively?
Do you have an uncomfortable feeling in your legs at night that causes you to move them around quite a bit? Or, does your bed partner report that you have excessive leg movement during sleep?
Do you generally feel rested when you wake in the morning?

If you have trouble falling or staying asleep, make sure you are practicing what is frequently called good "sleep hygiene." This means making sure you are avoiding any behaviors that could be interfering with your ability to fall asleep or stay asleep. Modifying such behaviors includes the following:

Minimize caffeine intake throughout the day, but especially after 2:00 or 3:00 P.M.
Minimize alcohol intake and definitely do not use it to help you fall asleep. If you do, you may wake up in the middle of the night or early morning as the alcohol wears off.
Avoid big meals right before bed so that your body is not busy digesting when it should be sleeping.

Use your bed to sleep in, not to get work done or to watch TV. Doing something stressful like catching up on work in bed does not create a restful climate. The bright lights of the TV right before bed may actually be causing you body to be in a more wakeful state and not ready to sleep.

If you cannot fall asleep after twenty or thirty minutes, get out of bed and do something in a dimly lit room that may make you fall sleepy. (Read a section of the newspaper that is not very appealing to you. Don't pick up your favorite book that you simply can't put down.)

Most of the above "sleep hygiene" recommendations are common sense, and many people who have had trouble sleeping have already made many of these changes. However, I chose to include the list just to make sure you feel that you have at least taken the basic steps toward better sleep before talking to your physician about a sleep medication.

I would never try to cover all of the medical reasons why someone may not sleep well at night. However, if you answered "yes" to some of the questions above, then you may have sleep problems that could readily be treated by a physician. An easy issue to address is the problem of getting up to use the bathroom too much at night. If you are not drinking a lot of fluid before bed, getting up more than once per night may indicate a treatable medical problem. Multiple sclerosis can cause a few different types of bladder problems, many of which can be helped with a medication before bed. Even without MS, men may experience increased nighttime bathroom trips as the prostate grows larger with age. Therefore, frequent sleep interruption due to trips to the bathroom is definitely something to discuss with your physician.

Other problems that can be related to MS are movement disorders of the legs or arms during sleep. "Restless Legs Syndrome" refers to an unpleasant feeling in the legs that results in the need to move the legs frequently in an attempt to become more comfortable. Patients are usually awake as they experience this and it prevents them from both falling asleep and staying asleep. Other patients have a problem that involves kicking and jerking their arms and legs intermittently throughout the night. This occurs more often when the person is sleeping, and it is frequently the bed partner who reports the symptom. Again, if you think these may be problems you are experiencing, your doctor can help you to achieve a better night's rest with a medication to decrease these symptoms.

Lastly, the diagnosis of "obstructive sleep apnea" (OSA) has received a great deal of press coverage over the past few years. Certainly, carrying extra weight increases a person's risk for this problem, but even thin people may have OSA. People suffering from sleep apnea frequently have very loud snoring and occasionally startle themselves awake. Despite having been in bed all night long and thinking they were sleeping, many people with OSA wake up feeling unrefreshed. For those diagnosed with sleep apnea, effective treatment can have a tremendous positive impact on quality of life as so much of the daytime fatigue resolves.

### Could Depression Be Causing Symptoms of Fatigue?

It is not unusual for those living with MS to experience depression at some point in time. If you have noticed a change in your overall mood, feel that tears come easily or have lost interest in many of your usual activities, you could be experiencing depression. Of course, if your diagnosis is still very new, a period of sadness and grieving is quite normal. However, if it has been several months since your diagnosis and persistent feelings of sadness or hopelessness are occurring, then it is probably time to talk to someone about possible depression. While we all think of mood changes as a sign of depression, fatigue can also be a symptom of depression. Some scientific studies suggest that treating depression in people with MS can result in improvement in symptoms of fatigue. This implies that for some people with MS, a part of their fatigue may in fact be coming from depression. Of course, if you suffer from severe fatigue, it may seem that the fatigue itself is causing you to feel depressed. If this sounds like a complicated case of "which comes first, the chicken or the egg," it very well can be.

When I was experiencing the daily fatigue I described earlier, I also began to experience occasional feelings of hopelessness. Tears began to come more easily. I was fairly certain that the symptoms of fatigue had come first. Still, I reached a point where I was not sure if the fatigue was causing some depressed feelings, or if the depression was beginning to contribute to increased fatigue. I felt pretty sure that my mood would improve if only I could regain my former levels of energy. I also knew that all this confusion about how I was feeling was an indication that it was time to speak to my doctor.

I raise the issue of depression in this chapter because it is a potential contributing factor to symptoms of fatigue. If you think you may be experiencing depression, getting assistance from your physician with medication and counseling may ultimately result in decreased symptoms of fatigue as well as improved mood and outlook. (Chapter 10 is devoted to the subject of depression and I encourage you to read it if you are at all concerned that you may be suffering from depression.)

### Are Medication Side Effects Contributing to My Fatigue?

In an earlier chapter, I emphasized the importance of getting on a current medication for multiple sclerosis as soon as possible after a diagnosis has been made. These are powerful medications that will likely decrease our rate of future relapses and may ultimately decrease the amount of disability we have. However, as we scrutinize all possible causes contributing to our fatigue, we must consider the fact that fatigue is a potential side effect of these medications. If a large part of your fatigue was felt to be coming from your MS medication, this would not mean stopping a disease-modifying drug altogether. Because there are several different medications available, you and your neurologist could discuss the option of trying a different one.

Sorting out whether fatigue is a result of your MS medication can be very challenging. I knew that before I had been diagnosed, I usually had enough energy to get through my busy days. It was not until approximately three years after my diagnosis that I began to experience midday waves of disabling fatigue. Was this new fatigue coming from the MS medication I had switched to several months earlier after the birth of my second child? Was I beginning to develop the primary fatigue that seems to come from MS itself? Or, was the challenge of having two children instead of one responsible for this fatigue?

In my case, I knew that I had lived almost three years with a diagnosis of multiple sclerosis with only mild fatigue. It seemed that something quite different had begun to happen in my body, causing these feelings of fatigue. Interestingly, after the birth of my second child, I had a severe allergic reaction to the disease-modifying medication I had taken before I became pregnant with her. Because of this new allergy, I had to change my MS medication. Although I had been on the new medication for many months before the fatigue really began to bother me, I was still suspect that it could be the culprit. Since the fatigue began to affect my quality of life and I felt that I was developing depression, my neurologist agreed it was time to try a medication switch again. Within two months of the change, those midday bouts of fatigue were nearly gone. My mood began to lift, and life began to look a lot better again.

I was very lucky to have such a good response to a change in medication. The majority of fatigue experienced in MS is not likely to be caused by the disease-modifying medications. As you try to decide whether your medication could be contributing to fatigue, an important question to ask yourself is whether you think the fatigue was something that truly began *after* you started taking your medication. Or, was there clearly a worsening of fatigue after the start of medication? Even if the answers to these questions are yes, changing medications right away is not necessarily the correct response. For many people, the side effects of flu-like symptoms and fatigue definitely decrease over time. If you have just started a medication that seems to be causing some fatigue, stick with the medication for a few months to see if your energy level improves before contemplating a change.

In addition to the possibility of the disease-modifying medications playing a role in fatigue, there are other drugs used for various symptoms in MS that may cause fatigue. Some of the medications used for bladder control, numbness and tingling, spasticity, or depression carry the possible side effect of fatigue. Asking the same questions about whether onset of the medication correlates with onset of your fatigue is important. Remember, we are fortunate to live at a time when there are many good medication options to treat various symptoms. Finding the right medication to control a particular symptom while minimizing the side effects can be challenging. There may be a period of trial and error until you find the right balance. However, I do believe that the balance can be found with a little patience and time.

### Is Heat Playing a Role in My Fatigue?

Fortunately, this is a straightforward question as we consider potential causes of fatigue. Just as heat can worsen chronic symptoms of MS such as numbness or weakness, heat can definitely increase fatigue. If I spend more than an hour outside in the heat of a North Carolina summer, I start to feel like a wet noodle. My arms and legs become heavy and floppy, and all my energy completely disappears.

If you live in a climate where the weather is particularly warm year round, the warm temperatures may be bringing about some fatigue. Of course, if you have access to an air-conditioned environment, the problem is readily solved. As long as you are able to keep cool, the outside temperatures are unlikely to affect you. For those who either work outside or do not have access to air-conditioning, the heat can become problematic. Various options such as fans, cooling vests, and cool drinks can be pursued if you are not readily able to escape the heat. For recreational time, keeping cool in a pool, lake, or ocean seems to help quite a bit while allowing you to remain outside.

### Am I Fatigued Because I Am "Overdoing It?"

Our society currently has everyone living at a fairly hectic pace. Every day, I speak to patients who feel like they are trying to be superhuman as they run around attempting to balance the stresses of work, family, finances, and more. While staying with your job or continuing to be an involved parent may be very important, a diagnosis of multiple sclerosis can serve as a wake-up call to seek ways to simplify some of the craziness.

I know that if I were to say yes to every opportunity to join a school or work committee, I would be exhausted trying to accomplish all the tasks that I had taken on. While I still have a very full and active life, my diagnosis has taught me that if I want to feel well, I have to know my own limits. If you are experiencing significant fatigue and feel that every day is a whirlwind tour of activities, look for ways to eliminate some of the activity. This may mean asking others for help at times. Or, it many mean not signing up for a certain committee next time. If you have a personality that has always taken on every possible task, making these changes may not be easy. But, if you are fatigued, you are probably struggling to do a good job with all of the tasks anyway. You will feel much better doing a good job on fewer tasks with less fatigue.

The ways in which we try to cut back on the hectic pace of our busy lives will be different for each of us. Yet, I do believe there are simple ways to decrease our fatigue every day. I have gone to a number of multiple sclerosis seminars and have read articles in which the speaker or author refers to "energy conservation techniques."[1] Most of the ideas I have heard over the years seem fairly obvious, but sometimes it is helpful to remind ourselves to strongly consider such options:

Plan your day around your energy highs and lows.

Be productive during the first few hours of the day.

If your schedule allows, take one to two short naps (no more than 30 minutes) or one long nap (45 minutes) each day when fatigue starts.

Plan for additional strenuous activities after a nap.

If napping is not an option with your current lifestyle, look for opportunities for a few ten-minute breaks throughout the day.

Plan your daily tasks at home or work in a manner that avoids extra trips from room to room, or up and down the stairs.

Sit for activities where sitting is an option.

When I look at such a list, it always seems to be in conflict with recommendations that tell us that regular exercise can help fatigue. On the one hand, we are being told to conserve our energy and to try to avoid doing physically demanding activities throughout the day. Yet, we are supposed to find time every day to make our bodies expend a good deal of energy as we exercise. Perhaps, the best way to think of it is that being constantly on the go all day long without any breaks creates a slow, continuous depletion of energy. A relatively short burst of exercise gets our metabolism going and causes release of certain chemicals in our body such as endorphins that may actually give us a little boost for the rest of the day. Regular exercise also results in a stronger body and greater endurance. When viewed from that perspective, it seems plausible that using energy conservation techniques throughout the day coupled with regular exercise may result in reduced fatigue.

## PRIMARY FATIGUE AND TREATMENT OPTIONS

By now, you have seen that it can take some real detective work to figure out which of many possible factors may be playing a role in the fatigue you experience as an individual living with MS. Many of these potential contributors such as sleep disorders or depression will require an intervention and some time before you know if your energy levels are going to improve. Once you feel that you have pursued and treated all possible causes of fatigue without improvement, then you may want to talk to your physician about treatment options for the primary fatigue of MS.

Of course many of the lifestyle interventions already mentioned above are very important in treating primary fatigue. The question that many want answered is whether or not there is a prescription medication that can decrease fatigue. Some of the medications that have been used over the years for patients with disorders such as narcolepsy have been studied for MS fatigue. Because scientific studies have not shown consistent results, using these medications for MS fatigue is sometimes controversial. Your best option is to speak with your physician so that he can assess your individual situation and make a recommendation as to whether or not a prescription medication for fatigue might be helpful for you.

## DON'T GIVE UP

Addressing all the questions in this chapter and attempting to figure out factors in your fatigue can seem overwhelming and exhausting in itself. The process of getting a handle on the causes of your fatigue followed by making lifestyle changes or starting treatments to help with the fatigue is going to take a good amount of time. An initial lifestyle change such as taking a daily nap may help, but not eliminate the problem. Making a second change such as trying a different medication for bladder problems may further decrease the fatigue.

Just as we have good days and bad days with our varied MS symptoms, we will have good and bad days with fatigue. If you have already had some fatigue as one of your MS symptoms, it may not be reasonable to expect that it will go away entirely. While I was fortunate to get rid of my midday wave of disabling fatigue by changing a medication, fatigue still pops up on different days in unpredictable ways. Weeks may go by as I run around with my busy life, and I may forget that I am even troubled by fatigue. Then, unexpectedly, I will experience a few days of feeling severely run down and tired for no apparent reason. When that happens, I start getting into bed a little earlier each night and try to practice more energy conservation techniques during the day. I try to listen to my body and give it the restful tune-up that it seems to be requesting.

If fatigue is having a significant impact on your daily quality of life, continue to seek solutions and to try different options. While they cannot see it, physicians who care for patients with MS know that our fatigue is real. They will try to help us as long as we keep trying to help ourselves. Don't give up.

# 10

# Could I Be Depressed?

Opening up to a chapter on depression is not an easy thing to do, especially if you feel you may be suffering from symptoms of depression. Finding motivation to do much of anything can be difficult when you are depressed. Or, perhaps, you are not certain whether you are experiencing true symptoms of depression, yet you know that you are not as emotionally balanced as you would like to be. I strongly encourage you to continue reading. Depression can negatively impact all aspects of your life—your relationships, your job, and your ability to take good care of yourself. Fortunately, you do not need to live with depression. There are many good options for help.

While you may not have known anyone else living with MS when you were diagnosed, you are certainly not alone if you are experiencing depressive symptoms. Depression affects between five and twenty percent of Americans in their lifetimes. For those living with MS, twenty-five to fifty percent of us will experience depressive symptoms at some point. Because mental health problems carry such a stigma in our society, many people are not willing to consider the possibility that they could be affected. In addition, it is often the person who is suffering from depression who is the least likely to recognize the symptoms. Many times, family, friends, or coworkers notice that a person has not "been himself" for a period of time before the individual with the depression begins to recognize this.

*I was just diagnosed with multiple sclerosis. Isn't it normal to feel sad?* As discussed in Chapter 2, it is very common at the time of diagnosis to go through a period of time marked by sad feelings and, perhaps, even hopelessness. For many, our self-image and sense of self-worth are challenged as we try to incorporate being "a person with multiple sclerosis" into the selves we have always known. This grieving process is both healthy and helpful as we work through the implications of the diagnosis in our lives. However, with the passage of time, there should be some healing and resolution of those sad feelings. We should reach a point where we feel ourselves moving forward. We should have the desire to get back to our regular activities. We should find ourselves laughing again and feeling happy when good things happen.

There is no defined time for how long the grieving process should last for any given person. However, a year is probably too long. Six months may even be too long if you have really withdrawn yourself from all your usual activities. During those first few weeks and months after diagnosis, there should be some sense that you are slowly but surely starting to feel better from an emotional standpoint. When the sad feelings never begin to lift, and feelings of hopelessness persist, then it is time to seek help for symptoms of depression.

Beyond that period of time when we are first diagnosed with MS and may be at risk for depression, symptoms of depression can still emerge at any point in the future. Sometimes, there may be a clear trigger for the onset of depressive symptoms such as a relapse of our MS or another significant life stressor. However, symptoms of depression can also surface without any clear reason for onset. These are the times that it may be particularly difficult to recognize the symptoms. Because there is a higher rate of depression in those living with MS, it is important to understand what is meant by "symptoms of depression."

## WHAT EXACTLY DO YOU MEAN BY "DEPRESSION"?

We all have a general sense of what the word "depression" means since it is used so commonly in our society. However, when doctors speak about "clinical depression" or "major depression," they are referring to a medical illness that is defined by a specific set of symptoms. Clinical depression is different from just having a down day because something did not go your way. When a person has a bad day, the feelings are usually temporary. She can still wake up the next day and go on with life. She is still capable of feeling very excited two days later when a good event happens. Those who are suffering from clinical depression have fairly persistent feelings of sadness. An event that should be perceived as very happy cannot suddenly lift the mood of the depressed person.

While I never want this book to read like a medical textbook, I decided to list the symptoms that are frequently used by physicians to make the diagnosis of depression. Because it is often difficult to recognize depressive symptoms in ourselves, reading through such a list may help to clarify what we are experiencing. Keep in mind that even within a formal diagnosis of depression, there are still degrees of severity. One person might technically meet the criteria, but the depth of her sadness or the extent of lost motivation may not be as great as another person's. Yet, even mild depression should not be ignored believing that it will eventually just go away. Many times it does not.

A diagnosis of depression can be made when a person has five or more of these symptoms on a daily basis:

Feeling sad or empty, or being irritable or tearful most of the day.
Loss of interest or pleasure in activities previously enjoyed.
Sleeping too much, or inability to sleep.
Decreased appetite and weight loss, or increased appetite and weight gain.
Restlessness, irritability.
Ongoing fatigue or loss of energy.
Difficulty concentrating or making decisions.
Feeling worthless, hopeless, or guilty without cause.
Thoughts of suicide or death.

## Is It Depression or MS?

In living with MS, sorting out depression from other symptoms that may be part of our illness can be quite confusing. Sleep problems, fatigue, and difficulty concentrating are all potential symptoms of MS, and yet they are on the list of symptoms of depression. The overlap of depressive symptoms with many other illnesses is part of the reason that strict criteria state that at least five symptoms from the list should be experienced on a daily basis to make a diagnosis of depression. In reality, I am not sure it is ever as simple as checking off symptoms from a list and saying yes or no regarding whether or not someone has depression.

In an earlier chapter, I described the way in which I lost the ability to sort out whether the fatigue I had was a symptom of depression, or whether I was starting to feel depressed because I was always so fatigued. When the picture gets confusing and you know you are not feeling yourself, it is best to seek help from your physician. An objective look at your symptoms from your neurologist who will be familiar with both symptoms of MS and depression may help to clarify your situation.

## What Depression Is Not

There are many misconceptions about depression in our society. Depression is not a weakness. It is not a defect in one's personality. It is also not something that you could make go away "if only you were a little stronger." You cannot "shake it off" or "ride it out." These are expressions I have heard many times from patients who waited a very long time before they sought help.

If we can let go of these negative notions of depression, we are more likely to pursue the assistance we need. While sorting out symptoms of depression from those of MS can be confusing at times, it is also important to realize that depression is likely to worsen one's perception of any existing MS symptoms. A chronic pain may begin to feel significantly worse in the setting of depression.

Certainly, one's ability to cope with the various challenges of MS will be diminished. We need to look past the stigma of depression so that we can maximize both our mental and physical health.

## WHY IS THERE AN INCREASED RATE OF DEPRESSION IN MS?

Some may think the answer to this question is obvious. People diagnosed with a chronic illness are going to experience more bouts of depression as a result of having to live with the illness. Yet, when researchers have tried to answer the question of why there is more depression in multiple sclerosis, living with a chronic illness does not seem to be the simple answer. One very interesting scientific study compared rates of depression in patients living with a number of different kinds of chronic medical conditions, including multiple sclerosis. Surprisingly, those living with MS still had higher rates of depression than those living with other chronic medical problems.[1] This type of finding causes many researchers to consider the possibility that there is something about the effect of MS on the brain that has the potential to cause depression.

When researchers or physicians discuss depression in patients with MS, they will sometimes identify the depression as being a primary, secondary, or tertiary depression. If the depressive disorder is felt to be a direct result of changes in one's brain from multiple sclerosis, it may be referred to as a primary depression. However, if there is a definitive cause of the depression such, as a side effect of medication, it may be referred to as a secondary symptom. Finally, depression may be called a tertiary effect if it stems from a particular situation such as changing family or job relationships as a result of living with MS. In reality, the source of someone's depression will not always fit neatly into any particular category. I share this terminology only because it may allow for a better appreciation of the various potential reasons for depression in MS.

## DEPRESSION AS A DIRECT RESULT OF MS

Is it possible that lesions occurring in certain areas of the brain could trigger symptoms of depression? At least two different scientific studies have looked at MRI brain scans of MS patients with and without depression. Both studies revealed that patients with depression did have specific areas of the brain that were more likely to show lesions than those who were not depressed.[2,3] However, there were some patients with MS who had lesions in those same brain areas that were not depressed. Therefore, it cannot be said with certainty that MS lesions occurring in particular areas of the brain are responsible for depression. Yet, these studies suggest that such changes in the brain may be a contributing factor.

As someone living with MS, I am slightly troubled in learning about a possible connection between brain lesions and depression. On the one hand, it is good to know that there may be a scientific explanation for higher rates of depression in MS. On the other hand, I do not want every person living with MS to conclude that he is definitely going to end up with depression at some point in time. It is important for us to be aware of depressive symptoms so that we might recognize them should they occur. However, a diagnosis of multiple sclerosis does not imply that future symptoms of depression are inevitable.

## DEPRESSION AS A POSSIBLE SIDE EFFECT OF MEDICATION

This is a subject area that is particularly challenging for me to discuss as someone who is both a patient with MS and a physician. Patients appropriately ask me about potential side effects when I prescribe a new medication for them. While I want my patients to be informed consumers, I do not want to set expectations for potential side effects just by mentioning them. I remind patients that the majority of possible side effects occur only in a minority of patients. If everyone taking the drug experienced a bothersome side effect, the drug likely would not have come to market. By raising the possibility that certain MS medications may have depression as a side effect, it is important to remember that most patients do not experience depression from the drugs. Yet, as a patient taking an MS medication, I certainly want to be aware of side effects that could impact my quality of life.

The scientific studies that suggest that depression may be a side effect from the interferon drugs used for the treatment of multiple sclerosis are not all in agreement. While some studies have shown higher rates of depression in patients on interferon therapy when compared to those taking a placebo medication,[4] other studies have not shown any difference in rates of depression between those taking interferon or a placebo.[5] The package inserts from the pharmaceutical companies of the three interferon medications list depression as a possible side effect. This means that depression was reported by a certain percentage of the patients taking the medication during the time when the companies were researching and developing the drugs. However, this does not prove a definite cause and effect.

It is critical that we do not use the first indication of a possible side effect from a medication as a reason to stop the drug right away. If you are on an interferon medication and you are experiencing symptoms of depression, it can be extremely challenging to sort out whether the depression is related to the use of the medication. Frequently, patients are beginning an interferon medication shortly after they have been diagnosed, a time when symptoms of depression may be forthcoming as a result of the new diagnosis. It may be easier to conclude that a drug is playing a role in depression if you were to change medications later in the course of your illness, and then develop symptoms of depression within a short period of time.

If you happen to be taking one of the interferon medications and think that you may be experiencing symptoms of depression, it is very important to discuss the symptoms with your physician. He may be able to help clarify whether or not the medication could be playing a role in your symptoms. Even when depressive symptoms are considered to be a possible medication-related side effect, these symptoms can readily be treated with safe and well-tolerated antidepressants. It is *so very important* that we find ways to stay on our disease-modifying therapy. There are times when this may mean taking a second medication to eliminate a side effect from the MS medication.

As mentioned earlier, I struggled for quite some time with symptoms of fatigue followed by mild depressive symptoms. Or, at least that was the order in which I thought the symptoms had occurred. As a physician, I kept trying to figure out what problem was causing which symptom. Was it MS that was causing me to feel fatigued? Or, was my medication causing me to feel fatigued? Was my excessive fatigue then making me depressed because my quality of life was not as good as I wanted it to be? Or, perhaps my medication was causing me to be depressed. If it sounds very confusing, it definitely was.

I eventually met with my physician, and we came up with a plan to try a few different strategies over the course of several months. Rather than starting an antidepressant while starting a medication for fatigue and switching my MS medication all at once, we decided to try one intervention at a time. In doing so, I could evaluate the effect of each change. It probably took nine months before I really felt "back to myself" again, but I did get there. Depression should be treatable, regardless of the underlying cause.

## DEPRESSION AS A RESULT OF LIFE CHANGES

Whether or not a person has developed a significant disability, a diagnosis of MS has the potential to place stress on our family relationships, our career, and other social interactions. When there is a physical or cognitive disability present, life stressors may be even greater as significant adjustments may need to occur in home, work, or social situations. There is already a challenge in maintaining our sense of self-worth as we learn that we have MS. If we then experience setbacks in relationships or career paths, symptoms of depression may be triggered.

If you are experiencing symptoms of depression and you can clearly identify some difficult changes in your family or work life since your diagnosis, this is a situation in which seeing a counselor may be particularly helpful. Antidepressant medication may still have an important role in this circumstance as well. For some, the combination of counseling and medication can be very effective when significant life changes have led to symptoms of depression.

## DISABILITY AND DEPRESSION

You may recall my earlier description of feeling like a coward as I sometimes look away from those with MS who have acquired significant disabilities.

Part of the reason for this is likely a natural reaction that comes from denial and self-preservation. I also know that I frequently make assumptions that those with substantial disabilities are not as happy as I am. Of course, this is a ridiculous assumption to make. Just because one's disease process has evolved to the point of a significant physical disability does not necessarily mean that the person cannot live a happy and fulfilled life. Perhaps, I make these assumptions because it would seem that social and vocational changes resulting from disability would more readily predispose these individuals to symptoms of depression.

Yet, studies do *not* consistently show that a person's level of disability correlates with rates of depression. A study mentioned earlier regarding higher rates of depression in patients with MS did suggest that depression occurred more often in patients with self-reported impairment or mobility limitations.[5] However, other studies that have looked for reasons for depression in patients with multiple sclerosis have not found that disability plays a role in rates of depression.[6]

It is important to keep in mind that these are scientific studies looking at large groups of people. They cannot predict how any one person will deal with his or her own disabilities. If and when a new disability comes along, there will inevitably be a period of adjustment. For some, it is certainly possible that the adjustment period may be more challenging and may serve as a trigger for depressive symptoms.

## VIEWING THE WORLD THROUGH A CLOUD OF DEPRESSION

Reading through an entire chapter on depression, especially if you feel that you may be experiencing symptoms of depression, can be a nearly impossible task. During the year that I was living with a combination of fatigue and depressive symptoms, I very likely would have stopped reading this chapter by now. I now describe that year as feeling like I was always waiting for the fog to lift. If you have come this far, I encourage you to finish the last few pages. It is important to identify steps you can take to get out from under that cloud of depression.

Viewing the world through a cloud of depression changes your perspective on all aspects of life. A depressed person takes less joy from the simple, every-day things such as your favorite team winning a big game, the sweetness of your favorite dessert, or a good joke shared with friends. A person suffering from depression also makes for a less giving partner or parent. Depression saps your energy and inclination for putting forth your best effort at work or school. Those who are depressed are also less likely to take interest in managing their MS.

Getting help with symptoms of depression means a better outcome not just for yourself, but for all those who are important to you in your life. If you do not have the motivation to get help for yourself, sometimes thinking about the impact of your depression on the loved ones in your life can provide the stimulus for you to take the first step.

## WHERE TO GO FOR HELP

There are many options in seeking help for symptoms of depression. Primary care physicians, neurologists, psychologists, and social workers will be knowledgeable in either helping you to treat your symptoms or directing you to a professional who can. For some of you, a close contact in a place of worship such as a minister or rabbi may feel like an easier place to start. Calling for an appointment in order to discuss such personal feelings can seem like a large hurdle to cross. Therefore, as you think about the professional you choose to discuss this with, your comfort level with that person may be one of the most important factors.

If you have always been a healthy person and don't feel like you have a comfortable relationship with any particular physician or trained professional, you should not let that stop you from pursuing assistance. In those situations, the neurologist who is treating your MS is a great place to start. Certainly, he will be very familiar with symptoms of depression in MS. He can then refer you to a counselor or another professional if he feels that this would be helpful in your particular case.

Even if your neurologist is not the first person you call to discuss symptoms of depression, it is important to let her know if you are being treated for depression. She may be able to help clarify some of the questions raised in this chapter about causes of depression in MS as it pertains to you as an individual. In addition, she should be aware of any antidepressant medication you may be taking. She may have some helpful thoughts about which antidepressant therapy could be best for you. There are some antidepressant medications that may have the added benefit of alleviating certain MS symptoms unrelated to depression. Other antidepressants have the potential to worsen particular symptoms of MS.

## TREATING DEPRESSION

While there is a stigma surrounding mental health disorders in our society that frequently prevents us from openly discussing such issues, I worry that the stigma regarding the use of medications to treat such problems is even greater. In living with MS, there may be several considerations as you contemplate the risks and benefits of taking a medication to treat symptoms of depression. First, many of us with MS may already be on a few different medications. The thought of adding the bother, expense, and potential side effects of yet another medication can be undesirable. Then, there is the very notion of "needing" a medication for depression. This is where our cultural and societal biases often come into play. Many people do not like the idea of being "dependent" on a medication for depression. Others feel like they are admitting some sort of weakness by taking antidepressant medication.

Hopefully, as you are coming to terms with living with MS, you are realizing that there are many different aspects to maintaining health and wellness. If taking an antidepressant for a period of time is what is needed to maintain your quality of life, then you need to view it as just one more thing you are doing to manage your health. In starting on a medication to treat depression, you are not signing on a dotted line to take it for the rest of your life. You and your physician will reevaluate your situation at various intervals and decide whether ongoing medication is needed. If you do start a medication, keep in mind that antidepressant medications are not one-type-fits-all. It may take a few trials until you find the medication that works best for you.

Seeking out help for symptoms of depression does not necessarily mean that an antidepressant medication will be recommended. Some individuals will find that regular counseling can be effective. Listen to the advice of the professional whose help you have sought. Remember that he or she has likely treated many others with similar symptoms and should have a good sense of what will be most helpful for you.

Last and very important, do not hesitate to talk to others living with MS about symptoms of depression. If you are in any sort of MS support group, or have met others with MS, these individuals can be a great resource for you. Some may be able to share ways they worked through a period of depression. Others who have not personally experienced depression can be guaranteed to lend a nonjudgmental and caring ear. It is part of what we share in this MS club.

## Hope

Those of us recently diagnosed with relapsing remitting MS have every reason to maintain hope for happy and fulfilling futures. In order for such futures to be realized, it is so very important that our emotional and mental health remains in good shape. Even if you are experiencing mild depressive symptoms, getting the right kind of help can dramatically change your outlook and your desire to make the most of whatever comes your way.

# 11

# YOU AND YOUR DOCTOR

I have said "talk to your physician" so many times in this book that I am afraid the physicians of the world will be wishing I did not write this book. Yet, in living with multiple sclerosis, your relationship with your physician is a key component in managing your health. You need to feel confident that your physician is knowledgeable about MS. You want to be sure that he keeps up to date with all the latest advances in treatment. Beyond having excellent medical knowledge, a physician who listens well will likely do a better job in making sure your concerns are being addressed.

Ideally, you also want your physician's office to have a support staff of nurses and assistants who can guide you through a number of different issues that may arise over the years: Can they help you if you experience problems with your injection medications? Can they assist you with insurance questions as you try to pay for expensive medications? Do they respond to your phone messages within a reasonable amount of time? All of this can sometimes sound like a tall order for a physician and his office staff. So what is considered reasonable to expect from the physician treating your MS? And, what can you do as a patient to improve your working relationship with your physician?

## WHO SHOULD BE MANAGING MY MS?

Before you think about how to make the most of your interactions with your physician, it is important that you believe you have found a physician who has experience in managing multiple sclerosis. As each of us went through the evaluation process that led to a diagnosis of MS, we probably went down a great many different paths, seeing many different types of physicians. Some of you may have been referred to a neurologist who ultimately made the diagnosis. Others who experienced optic neuritis may have had an ophthalmologist tell you that you have MS. Some may have had their internist or family doctor make the diagnosis.

If you were not initially diagnosed with MS by a neurologist, then you were probably referred to one for treatment recommendations and long-term management. Many times, patients will ask if there are neurologists who specialize in treating MS. It is true that even within the field of neurology, physicians frequently subspecialize to treat different types of illnesses within the neurology specialty. If you live in a large city, or in a town where there is a medical school, there are probably several neurologists who focus on the treatment of specific neurological illnesses. In this case, your primary care physician may be a good resource who knows whether there are neurologists in your area that specialize in the treatment of MS.

On the other hand, if you live in a smaller city or town, there may not be a neurologist who focuses mainly on the treatment of multiple sclerosis. However, this should not be a cause for concern on your part. In these situations, the general neurologists usually have an excellent ability to treat and manage MS because they are the ones caring for the patients with MS in their communities. They will also be aware of MS experts in your larger region and can always refer you to one of these subspecialists if they think it would provide additional benefit.

If you have questions about a particular physician's familiarity in treating MS, there are many different ways to learn more about that physician. Many medical offices now have on-line Web sites where you can read a small biography about each of the physicians. In addition to telling you where a particular physician went to medical school and did his training, these biographies frequently tell you about the physician's area of expertise in treating patients. Your local chapter of the National MS Society is also an excellent resource for a listing of neurologists in your area who care for patients with MS.

I realize that this may sound like quite a bit of "homework" to do in order to find a neurologist to help manage your MS. If you are already very satisfied with your current neurologist, then there is no reason to pursue other options. However, if you feel that your current physician does not have a lot of experience in treating MS, then it is worth spending the time to find someone who does.

Although I was working at a major academic medical center when I was diagnosed, I did not have the confidence I needed in the neurologist who had ordered my MRI. He had expertise in other areas of neurology, but he had not treated MS patients in many years. So even though it was somewhat awkward, I switched my care to a different neurologist who had many MS patients in her practice.

## WORKING WITH YOUR NEUROLOGIST

As someone who has spent a good amount of time being both the physician and the patient, I truly consider the patient–physician relationship to be a partnership in which each member has distinct tasks and responsibilities. Your neurologist has the very important job of determining which disease-modifying medication will work best for you as an individual to minimize future MS relapses while causing the fewest side effects. Part of her role is to help educate you about these disease-modifying therapies and to help you understand why she is recommending a particular one for you. In addition to prescribing a medication to decrease the frequency of relapses, your neurologist is the one who can treat many of the symptoms of MS that can emerge, such as fatigue, numbness and tingling, bladder difficulties, or depression.

Beyond being competent in treating MS and its various symptoms, there are many other qualities that we desire in our physician. If your neurologist is going to be able to sort through the sometimes confusing symptoms of MS, then she needs to provide the opportunity for you to explain whatever it is that you are experiencing. While she may have several specific questions for you about other symptoms that enable her to clarify your situation, it is important for you to feel that your concerns have been conveyed and heard.

Of course, the physician cannot be entirely responsible for the success of your partnership with him. As patients, we do not always consider ourselves to have an active role to play in our physician–patient relationship. Yet, there are definitely a few simple steps we can take as patients to get the most from a visit with our neurologists. As a starting point, taking a few minutes to prepare for your visit can be very beneficial. If there are certain symptoms or concerns that you want to be sure are addressed, consider writing down them down so that you are not suddenly raising a forgotten concern at the end of a visit. In my role as a physician, patients occasionally apologize to me if they show up at a visit with a list of concerns. I tell them that I never mind reviewing a list with them as long as we are both reasonable about what can be covered during that visit. When patients have written down their concerns, it sends a message to me that they have taken the visit seriously, and it helps me know what to focus on during that encounter.

As you discuss issues with your physician, it is critical that you are honest about what has been taking place. Many of you may think, "Well of course I am honest with my doctor. Why wouldn't I be truthful with my doctor?" Sometimes patients may *stretch* the truth a bit because they want to be perceived as a "good patient." For example, if you have been taking a medication only a few times per week that is supposed to be taken every day, your doctor needs to know this. Otherwise, your physician may conclude that the medication is not working for you, when in fact you are not taking it very often. He also needs to know why you may not be taking a medication as recommended. If there are side effects from the medication, he may be able to recommend a method to alleviate the side effects. If the cost of your medication prevents you from regular use, he needs to know this too. There may be a patient assistance program that enables you to get your medication at a lower cost.

As you sit and discuss concerns with your physician, remember that doctors are not mind readers. While they may try very hard to ask open-ended questions and give you a chance to share what is on your mind, they may still overlook something that has been bothering you. This tends to happen more often with issues that we consider to be of a "personal" nature, such as difficulties with functioning of bladder, bowels, or sexuality. Therefore, if you have such concerns and your neurologist has not specifically asked you about them, it is important for you to bring these problems to his or her attention. Keep in mind that neurologists who care for patients with MS discuss these types of "personal" issues many times each day. They will discuss such concerns with you in a professional manner and will be able to provide you with treatment recommendations.

As you and your doctor work to find medications that are best for you, remember that no two people will have exactly the same response to a particular medication. If it turns out that a medication has not been effective for you, or if you experience an unpleasant side effect, this does not mean that your physician has made a bad decision about treatment for you. Realize that whether you are beginning a new disease-modifying medication or a medication to treat a particular symptom, it may occasionally require a few trials of different medications to find the one that is the right fit for you. When you are seeking relief from a bothersome symptom, it can be very challenging to be patient as new medications are being tried. When you meet with your physician after trying a new medication, be specific about any improvements you have noticed as well as any side effects you may have had. This allows your physician to fine-tune your medications for maximum benefit to you.

I have emphasized the importance of open communication between you and your physician. One of the challenges for both the patient and the physician is communicating all of the important information in a defined period of time. Unfortunately, physicians do not have the leisure of spending one or two hours with each patient they see. While many of them would like to be able to have that much time for each visit, they would never be able to accommodate all the patients who need their expertise. Therefore, it is also helpful to prioritize your list of concerns when you go for an appointment. If you are unable to cover all the issues in a single visit, then you can address the concerns that were lower on your list at the next visit. You may also want to think about which members of your physician's office staff can assist with some of your concerns that are not directly related to medical symptoms. For example, nurses will be able to instruct you about how and when to take medications. Other office personnel may be able to assist with insurance questions, referrals to physical therapy, or names of support groups in town.

## WHAT ABOUT PHYSICIANS BESIDES MY NEUROLOGIST?

If you went to a primary care physician up until the time of your diagnosis, then he or she will still be the doctor you go to for much of your health care. Most doctors who identify themselves as "primary care physicians" have trained as either internal medicine physicians or as family medicine physicians. After a diagnosis of MS, your primary care physician is still the one you would see for regular "checkups" that include preventive care services such as cholesterol and blood pressure checks as well as recommendations for various screening tests such as mammograms or colonoscopy. Your primary care physician is also the one you will still see you for "acute illnesses" such as the flu, other infections, or an injury. Some primary care physicians will also be able to play a role in the management of MS symptoms or medication side effects.

In living with multiple sclerosis, there will be many times when you are uncertain about whether a new symptom is related to your MS or not. If you experience a new symptom for one to two days that you feel may be related to your MS, it is always worthwhile to call your neurologist's office. Your neurologist or her nurse can then make a recommendation as to whether the symptom should be evaluated right away in their office, or whether they would like you to see your primary care physician first. Your primary care physician will factor your MS into his evaluation so that he can assist in sorting out what may be causing a particular symptom.

Beyond maintaining your relationship with your primary care physician, there may be other physicians that you meet over the years who will assist in the management of your MS. While your neurologist will treat the majority of issues that arise in relationship to your MS, there may be times when she recommends another specialist to further evaluate a particular symptom. For example, if you were to have problems with vision, your neurologist may refer you to an ophthalmologist who has experience in treating visual disorders associated with MS. If you were to experience bladder problems that did not respond to typical medications, a urologist would be the type of specialist that could offer some additional advice. Physicians who specialize in the field of physical medicine and rehabilitation may be particularly helpful with problems related to gait, strength, or balance.

Thinking about the possibility of seeing so many physicians can be overwhelming. For most of you, the majority of your doctor visits over the next several years will likely be with either your neurologist or your primary care physician. Yet, it is helpful to realize that there may be times when another specialist can provide additional insight and recommendations about a particular problem you may be having. If your neurologist has recommended that you see a specialist, it is because he believes that that type of physician can be of additional assistance to you.

Earlier this year, I began to experience a significant increase in the pain in both of my eyes. The pain was very similar to what I had experienced thirteen years ago with my optic neuritis. Although I was not having any definite visual symptoms, I was convinced that I had optic neuritis again. My neurologist did a thorough eye exam and ran some visual tests in his office. He did not think it was optic neuritis, but he knew how concerned I was. He referred me to a neuro-ophthalmologist who reassured me that there was no evidence of active optic neuritis. I was very relieved and did not mind having made the trip to another physician's office.

## OTHER MEDICAL PROBLEMS

Many of you who are newly diagnosed with MS are young, in your twenties or thirties. You may not have any other significant medical problems that require regular doctor visits or treatment. If this is the case, then seeking ways to stay fit and healthy as discussed in Chapter 8 will hopefully become a priority for you. However, if you had other medical problems before the diagnosis of MS, such as diabetes or high blood pressure, then it is critical that you continue to see the physicians who help to manage those illnesses as well. The course of your MS is likely to be better when any other medical problems are kept under good control.

If you have other medical problems in addition to MS, keeping up with a number of different physicians may become time-consuming, tiring, or financially challenging. Many of your other problems may already be managed by your primary care physician. However, if you have always gone to a number of different specialists, talk to your primary care physician about what he can help you to manage. Your primary care doctor may be able to assist in the treatment of some of your other medical problems that would enable you to decrease the frequency with which you see other specialists. However, be sure to talk to your primary care physician about what he feels is best before concluding that you are going to decrease the number of visits to another physician. There are some medical problems for which it is always best to have a specialist involved on a regular basis.

## AN IMPORTANT RELATIONSHIP

Because you will be managing your MS for a lifetime, it is important that you have a good working relationship with your neurologist. When I go to an appointment with my neurologist, I always feel that I have his full attention and that he carefully listens to what I have to tell him. He explains to me any new treatment options he may be considering, and he tells me why he would consider them in my particular situation. While there may be times when I do not feel ready to try something new or different, I know that he makes such recommendations because he is truly considering what is best for me. Some may think that I get "extra attention" from my neurologist because I am also a physician. However, I am certain from speaking to other patients who see him that he gives every one of his patients the same amount of time and careful thought that I receive.

I know I am fortunate to have found an excellent neurologist. I also know that there are many other outstanding neurologists who treat patients with MS. As you seek to establish a relationship with a neurologist, it is very reasonable to expect to feel a level of comfort and confidence that is similar to what I experience with my physician. Yet, keep in mind that just like the development of any other working relationship, it may take several visits before you might actually use the word "comfortable" to describe the way you feel in your neurologist's office. After all, if given a choice, most of us would rather not have a reason to be there in the first place. Hopefully, given that you do have reason to see a neurologist, you will eventually come to believe that you have found the right one.

## LEARNING TO BE A PATIENT

If you are still adjusting to a recent diagnosis, you may not have any desire to seek out a neurologist and to work on establishing a good patient–physician relationship. You may not be ready to think about seeing any physician on a regular basis. You did not ask to be a patient.

Physicians are certainly aware of these potential feelings. Therefore, just getting yourself to the necessary appointments during the first six months may be all that you seek to accomplish as a patient. As with many of the issues that arise with a diagnosis of MS, *give yourself time* to adjust to your role as a patient. When you are ready to share additional concerns or ask more questions, your physician will be there to listen.

# 12

# DEALING WITH DISABILITY

When facing a diagnosis of MS, the word *disability* has the potential to elicit more anxiety than the words *multiple sclerosis* do. The thought of ever becoming disabled is the very thing we fear when we are told we have MS. During the first few years after my diagnosis, I slowly came to accept the fact that I had MS and it was here to stay. Yet, I still had some very strong denial mechanisms taking place when it came to the "D" word. Although I had several invisible symptoms like numbness, fatigue, and episodic dizziness, I never would have considered myself to be disabled.

If I had been reading a book such as this when my diagnosis was still relatively new, I probably would have skipped this chapter because I would have felt that it was not relevant to my situation. Perhaps you are wiser than I was at the time and you have chosen to read this chapter so that you are well informed about all aspects of living life with multiple sclerosis, whether or not you presently have any significant impairment. If you do have new symptoms that are creating some limitations for you, then it is my hope that this chapter will provide both encouragement and resources for dealing with whatever your particular situation may be.

## DEFINITIONS

Using the word *disability* in any given situation depends on how you choose to define the word. In our society, the word *disability* commonly refers to a type of physical impairment that limits the usual activities of an individual. It can imply that a person will need to make some adaptations in the ways he accomplishes specific tasks in order to remain an active participant in society. We frequently think of an individual with a disability as having the need to use some type of assistive device such as a brace, walker, or scooter. These would certainly be appropriate descriptions of the concept of disability. However, disability can also result from problems that are not purely physical. Problems with short-term memory or finding the right words are examples of cognitive impairments that can cause challenges in everyday living. Severe fatigue or inability to stay out in the heat may create "disabilities" for individuals whose situations do not allow for naps or a cool, indoor environment.

The World Health Organization (WHO) uses the word *impairment* in the same context that the word *disability* is often used. Impairment can be defined as "a problem in a body system or body part that significantly deviates from the norm."[1] Coming up with a precise definition for disability or impairment may not seem very important if you are the one experiencing the limitation. After all, you will know exactly what the word impairment means in your own situation. However, I believe that if we are going to be educated patients, then we should try to have some familiarity with the different words that may used by both the health care profession as well as by governmental agencies to describe physical or cognitive limitations.

Specific disability scales that rate the level of an individual's disability are sometimes used by physicians to track a patient's progress. More commonly, the scales are used in MS research studies as a means to provide objective data about the disability level of the participants in the studies. Beyond defining disability with numerical scales for medical purposes, the word disability takes on a very detailed definition when criteria are being assessed to determine whether or not a person qualifies for social security disability insurance (SSDI; to be discussed later in this chapter.)

## COMING TO TERMS WITH OUR OWN DISABILITIES

While I made reference to the "D" word in terms of my own initial feelings of denial about potential disability, this type of attitude is ultimately not helpful for any of us. Yet, I would not expect anyone to easily accept the idea of "having a disability." In the beginning, we are still trying to come to terms with the diagnosis of MS at the same time that we may be recovering from whatever symptoms led to the diagnosis. We have been told that we have "relapsing–remitting MS." Therefore, we anxiously await the remission of those symptoms as the name of the illness implies.

Within several months of our diagnosis, we will probably have a good feeling for whether or not there are going to be any long-lasting physical, sensory, or cognitive impairments. If we do have symptoms that persist, the way in which these symptoms impact our everyday functioning will create our own personal perception of whether or not we now have some type of disability. Even though I lost my ability to spin without getting terribly sick, I never considered this to be a disability because spinning is not something I need to be doing.. When I realized I could not stay out in the heat for very long, this was also not a disability in my mind because I always have the option of returning inside. However, if I had not recovered the vision in my left eye after my episode of optic neuritis, surely I would have considered that to be a disability.

There are many inspiring stories in the MS literature about the ways in which individuals have overcome or compensated for a particular disability. If you are dealing with a new impairment, you may find it very encouraging to read some of these stories. But if you are not ready to hear about others' triumphs when you are still struggling with your own new challenges, then your focus should be on finding out what you need to do in order to keep moving forward. The goal for all of us with MS should be to remain active and engaged members in our homes and communities, no matter what may come our way.

## Physical Disabilities

### "Will I Be in a Wheelchair Someday?"

This is the unspoken thought that comes to mind for so many of us when first diagnosed. It is the belief in our current era of disease-modifying medications that the majority of us with relapsing–remitting MS (RRMS) will *not* have the need for a wheelchair someday. The older, frequently reported statistics that states that half of people with RRMS will need some assistance with walking within fifteen years of diagnosis does not reflect the introduction of the newer medications. However, even if a wheelchair is less likely to be in our futures, we still need to recognize that there will likely be some type of impairment along the way that requires some adaptation to the way we do things.

The first time we ever have to deal with a physical disability can feel like a tremendous setback in so many ways. There is the actual physical impairment itself that may present a whole new set of challenges. Then, there is the accompanying emotional upset when we may begin to feel like "the MS is winning." With RRMS, there is also the psychological challenge of not knowing if a new physical impairment that occurs in the setting of a relapse is going to be temporary or long-lasting. Will there be partial recovery or complete recovery? If a degree of weakness remains after an exacerbation, will it slowly get worse over the years?

Only time can answer such difficult questions. Even though I described some of my MS symptoms that I never considered to be significant impairments, I still had to make some minor adjustments along the way to accommodate for these symptoms. As much as I used to love the spinning rides at an amusement park, I now choose to sit out and watch my husband and children on those rides. The vertigo and nausea I would experience should I choose to ride would stay with me for hours. This is certainly not a big deal since we don't go to amusement parks very often. But there are times when I do feel somewhat disabled when a simple game of "ring-around-the-rosy" or swinging on a park swing can leave my head spinning. Sometimes, I feel trapped in my air-conditioned house as I watch my kids run around outside on hot summer days, knowing that I would feel like a limp piece of lettuce if I joined them for more than a few minutes.

These are examples of very minor impairments with ready solutions. There are countless games to play with my children that do not involve spinning.

During the summer, I spend most of my time outside with my children in the pool where I can stay cool. Interestingly, however, in the course of writing this book, I have begun to develop a new physical disability with my right arm. While I have had some chronic numbness and tingling in my right arm since my diagnosis in 2000, I have had increasing feelings of heaviness and weakness in my right arm in the previous six months. These symptoms developed during the same year that I switched to a new job that involved hand-writing the majority of patient notes rather than dictating notes while also spending my evenings typing on a computer to complete a book. Therefore, for the first time since I was diagnosed with MS, I have found myself having to make some specific adjustments in how I complete tasks on a daily basis because of a mild physical impairment.

### "So What Do We Do When a Physical Disability Comes Along?"

After having had this recent experience with my arm, I believe the most important thing we can do is to pursue the necessary assistance to ensure that we can continue to participate in our home and work life to whatever our fullest capacity may be. The extent to which we are able to continue participation will depend on the particular physical disability and its impact on our usual activities at home or work. Had I been a surgeon, the heaviness in my arm might have limited my ability to fully participate in my profession. As an internist, there were several different types of interventions I was able to pursue to prevent my arm symptoms from slowing me down.

Interventions to help with a physical disability can come in many different forms including the use of assistive devices or adaptive technology, creating workspace accommodations, or taking part in physical or occupational therapy. Terminology such as "assistive devices" and "adaptive technology" may sound somewhat foreign if you are newly encountering a disability. Applied to my particular situation, I decided that writing numerous patient notes throughout my workday was contributing to the weakness and fatigue of my arm muscles. Therefore, the "adaptive technology" I acquired was a handheld dictaphone so that I no longer had to write any patient notes. Through the advice of an occupational therapist, I learned that the simple "assistive device" of a rubber grip on my pen would decrease the strain on my hand muscles during the times that I did write. Lastly, I acquired an ink stamp of my signature so that I could decrease the number of times I have to sign my name throughout the day.

### But What if MS Affects My Ability to Walk?

The unspoken fear of being in a wheelchair someday stems from the fact that many different symptoms of MS can impact one's ability to walk. Not only do weak or tight muscles contribute to gait (walking) problems, but changes in sensation, balance, or vision all have the potential to create difficulties with walking. Once symptoms do begin to occur that interfere with one's ability to walk, some individuals may take the approach of avoiding certain situations in order to avoid dealing with the gait problem. Others may put off using an assistive device, such as a cane, for as long as possible. There is no doubt that using a cane or a walker makes a disease that may have previously been invisible to others suddenly seem very visible. Resistance to the use of such aids or even to participating in a physical therapy program is a very normal reaction. Not only do these things make the disease more visible to others, but there is a feeling of being defeated by the disease.

It is important to try to "turn the tables" on this disease when we face a new disability that is as frightening as a change in the way we walk. Rather than feeling defeated by the disease, we need to muster up the emotional strength to get ourselves to pursue the help we need. The way in which we react to a disability greatly affects the degree to which that disability negatively impacts our lives. Avoiding physical therapy can result in further loss of muscle strength rather than maintaining or even restoring some function. Being resistant to the use of an assistive device may mean sitting out from an activity in which participation could otherwise have taken place. If we were to allow a gait disturbance to keep us from going places that we have always enjoyed, then we may find ourselves not only struggling with a new physical disability, but we may begin to experience sadness over the loss of social interaction.

In living with MS for a lifetime, it is critical that we do not let physical impairments "take us out of the game." Both our mental and physical health will be better if we discover ways to remain active in our homes, communities, and work lives.

## So Where Do We Go for Help with a Physical Disability?

A medical specialty called "Physical Medicine and Rehabilitation" comprises a team of professionals who come together to assist patients with a variety of physical and cognitive problems. These teams may consist of physicians (sometimes called "physiatrists"), physical therapists, occupational therapists, speech therapists, and neuropsychologists. If you live in a large city or town, there may be an entire Department of Physical Medicine and Rehabilitation located in a major medical center. Even without a major rehabilitation center nearby, all cities and town will have locations providing rehabilitation services for those with MS.

If you are newly diagnosed, the idea of needing "rehabilitation" may seem a bit extreme. "Do I really need to go for rehabilitation? My leg is just a bit weak." Many of us think of rehabilitation as something people do after a major car accident or a major surgery. Others may relate the term only to centers for drug and alcohol rehabilitation. It is definitely easier to say that you are going to look into "physical therapy" options since most people are familiar with that term. Yet, I have chosen to introduce you to the broader field of physical medicine and rehabilitation because it encompasses many different services in addition to physical therapy that may be helpful for you.

As an example, an individual experiencing some mild leg weakness may begin by working with a physical therapist. But if that person was also tripping a lot, a physiatrist or physical therapist may recommend that a foot device be worn to prevent the tripping. If that same person happened to drive a car for a living, then an occupational therapist could assist him with adaptive technology that might enable him to keep driving with a weak leg.

When you are ready to initiate a therapy or rehabilitation program, your neurologist or his or her staff should be able to guide you in finding the appropriate physical and occupational therapy centers in your area. Frequently, your neurologist will be the one who first suggests that you participate in some type of therapy program. If there are physicians in your town who specialize in the field of rehabilitation, there may be times when your neurologist recommends a consultation with one of them. Rehabilitation physicians have expertise in identifying problems with specific body "mechanics" and can help to tailor a therapy program that is best for your specific needs. If you are interested in learning more about what the field of rehabilitation medicine can offer, there is a wonderful brochure produced by the National Multiple Sclerosis Society (NMSS) called "Managing MS through Rehabilitation." It can be found in the NMSS Web site library or you can mail order it to your home.

## WHAT IF I AM HAVING PROBLEMS WITH MEMORY OR THOUGHT PROCESSES?

When most of us think about disability, we think about problems with the way we walk, talk, see, or use our hands. We think about physical problems that are sometimes referred to as problems with "motor function." However, problems with cognition, or the way we think, may be present in up to half of the people living with MS. This is another one of those MS statistics that I don't like to hear. While the majority of us may fear the thought of being in a wheelchair someday, most of us probably fear the loss of our cognitive abilities even more. As with all other MS symptoms, the degree to which cognitive problems are experienced will vary greatly from person to person.

So what specific types of problems are considered to be cognitive impairments? Problems with memory, difficulty learning new information, or decreased speed of processing information are all examples of cognitive problems that may occur in MS. Just as it is sometimes difficult to determine whether or not a physical symptom we are having is due to our MS, it may be even harder to determine if a cognitive problem is due to our MS. Many of us have had the experience of running into someone at the grocery store that we just met at a social event one week ago, and we cannot begin to remember the person's name. Or, we may walk into a room in our home to get a particular item and then we are not sure what we had come to get once we are in the room. If these types of things happen once in a while, should we worry that we are having cognitive problems stemming from multiple sclerosis? Not necessarily.

In our hectic, overscheduled, multitasking society, I frequently hear many of my healthy patients in their thirties or forties describing these very same types of memory lapses. Therefore, an occasional memory lapse probably does not deserve further attention. However, if you find yourself experiencing these types of memory lapses several times each week, and it seems to be a change from your baseline, then it is appropriate to discuss your concerns with your neurologist. Other examples of cognitive problems include difficulty completing tasks at home or work in the same time frame previously accomplished, getting mixed up while performing a task you have done many times, such as preparing your favorite dish, or forgetting to complete tasks of greater consequence, such as turning off the stove after cooking. Sometimes, it may be your family members or significant others who notice these types of problems before you do.

If you have *any* concerns that you may be experiencing impairment in your memory or thought processing, be sure to provide specific examples of situations where you have noticed a problem to your neurologist. He will likely ask a number of questions to help sort out the extent of the problem and to determine whether or not other issues such as a sleep disorder, depression, or fatigue could be playing a role in your cognitive changes. If one of these other factors were to exist, such as poor sleep quality, it would be important to treat the sleep disorder first and monitor the impact on your cognitive function.

Occasionally, your neurologist may refer you to a neuropsychologist who will be able to define the precise nature of the difficulties you are having with your memory or thought processing. I realize that the professional title of "neuropsychologist" can sound very intimidating and may cause someone to decide that perhaps the memory problems are not so bad after all. However, a consultation with such a professional can provide great insight for both you and your neurologist. Through a series of questions, a neuropsychologist can help to pinpoint which aspects of memory or thought processing are most difficult for you. He or she will also be able render an opinion as to whether your cognitive difficulties are most likely resulting from MS versus another problem such as depression.

## Are Problems with Cognition Considered to Be a Disability?

Just as with any physical impairment, problems with cognition may become a disability for an individual when they begin to interfere with successful completion of everyday tasks. I met a woman in her forties at an MS conference whose previous career had involved a type of investigative work. Initially, she had continued to work full time after her diagnosis, and she considered herself to be very fortunate because she did not have any significant physical impairments. However, one day when she was driving alone in her car, she found herself feeling lost in a neighborhood that was very familiar to her. She had to call her husband to bring her home. Of course, this episode frightened her tremendously. At the conference, she discussed the fact that, in retrospect, she had been having some other problems with cognition prior to her episode of getting lost. However, life had been busy and she never thought to discuss the problems with her neurologist. For this woman who had been working as an investigator, her cognitive impairments caused a significant limitation in her ability to perform her job.

### Where Do I Go for Help with Cognitive Problems?

If your neurologist has referred you to a neuropsychologist in order to better define the nature of your cognitive difficulties, then the neuropsychologist can also assist in developing a therapy plan. Frequently, the actual therapy is done with an occupational therapist. Therefore, there may be circumstances when your neurologist chooses to refer you directly to an occupational therapist. When your problems are with short-term memory, the "therapy" may come in the form of designing strategies to compensate for poor memory such as list making, use of handheld computers, or even maximizing cell phone capabilities. If your problems are with learning or thought processing, an occupational therapist will have many different resources not only to help you compensate for the specific problems but to "train your brain" to maximize your existing abilities.

## OTHER TYPES OF DISABILITIES

Problems with motor function and cognition are not the only types of disabilities that those living with MS may experience. Impairment in vision, speech and language, or bladder and bowel function all have the potential to cause disability. In addition, severe fatigue, or painful sensory changes can cause substantial disability. Reading a list of potential disabilities as someone living with MS can be quite disheartening. Yet, the take-away message is that there is an entire medical specialty devoted to improving and maintaining function for all of these different types of problems. There are rehabilitation specialists and therapists who can assist with the spectrum of motor, sensory, and cognitive impairments. In our current era, there is also a vast array of incredible technology to help with many different problems.

## WHAT IF I NEED TO CONSIDER APPLYING FOR SOCIAL SECURITY DISABILITY INSURANCE (SSDI) BENEFITS?

Before you take the step of applying for SSDI benefits, I would encourage you to explore all possible avenues with either your current job or within a similar line of work. While I will never know the unique situations of each person reading this book, I do believe that many benefits come from staying active in a job beyond the obvious financial ones. Chapter 6 discusses in detail many of the questions to be considered when trying to decide what is best for your personal situation. Whether you want to try to stay in your current job or to find alternative work that may better fit with your current abilities, a "vocational rehabilitation specialist" will be able to help. At times, there may be ready solutions in your current work environment by making certain accommodations or adaptations. Alternatively, a vocational specialist can assist you with retraining for a different type of position if that were a better option for you.

With that having been said, there may come a time when applying for SSDI benefits is the right course of action for you to take. While I have neither personal experience nor professional expertise in this area, I have heard from others with MS as well as from many of my own patients that the benefits application process can be a long and frustrating path. This should not be a reason to avoid pursuing benefits if it is clearly the right decision for you. But it will require that you educate yourself as well as you can before you undertake the process. You should also strongly consider seeking out assistance from someone who has some experience in the area. As a starting point, the National Multiple Sclerosis Society has a link on their Web site that can guide you through the application process (nationalmssociety.org/SSDI). The Social Security Administration (SSA) should also have representatives available either in person or on the phone to assist with questions.

The SSDI application process can be challenging for many different reasons. First, and somewhat discouraging to hear, is the statistic from the NMSS that almost half of the people with MS applying for SSDI are denied at least once before being accepted. This means that you need to be ready for the possibility of having to go through an appeals process. Therefore, you also need to be prepared for the possibility that it may be well over a year from the day that you complete the application process until the day that you actually begin to receive benefits.

The other major challenge in the application process is actually proving that you meet the criteria to receive benefits. A qualifying disability is considered a permanent impairment. Given the waxing and waning nature of MS symptoms, this can sometimes be difficult to prove. In addition, a person has to be incapable of performing any kind of work, not just the job she had previously held. Arguments could be made that a person with a physical disability who had previously worked as a dance instructor could learn to do a desk job. An accountant with cognitive impairments affecting her computing abilities might still be able to do a job that is less mentally demanding.

There is a list of precise disability requirements that can be obtained from the SSA office or from their Web site (see "Resource" section). In all likelihood, your neurologist will be familiar with the requirements, but you should plan to provide him with a printout of the SSA requirements so that he may document your symptoms appropriately. Your neurologist may also have enough experience with other patients who have gone through the application process to provide you with an opinion on how well your specific situation meets the SSA requirements.

If you believe that pursuing SSDI benefits is the right course of action, then you should not give up in your pursuit. I know I am not providing great words of encouragement when it comes to the process. It is important for you to have realistic expectations of what the process entails. However, if up to half of people are denied at least once before getting benefits, there is another half who receives benefits after the first application. For those who do get denied the first time, there are many resources available to assist with the appeals process.

## DEALING WITH DISABILITY

Although I have come a long way in my approach to thinking about my own potential disabilities in living with MS, I am still human and do not like to spend too much time contemplating such possibilities. I do feel fairly confident that current disease-modifying drugs will decrease the degree of disability that is seen over the long run in individuals diagnosed with multiple sclerosis in this era. Yet, I need to be realistic and acknowledge that many individuals with RRMS will still experience some type of impairment over time, even if relatively minor.

Whether we view a disability that we may have as minor or severe, it is critical that we seek out the assistance we need to ensure that we remain active participants in all of the things that life has to offer. Allowing ourselves to become isolated would only lead to a decline in our emotional health, with a subsequent decline in our overall health. Seek out the help from physical and occupational therapists in order to minimize the impact of a disability on your home or work life. Do what you can to maintain or improve muscle strength, cognition, or speech. While potentially unappealing at first, consider the use of assistive devices or adaptive technology as recommended by your therapist. You may be surprised to find out how liberating such devices can be.

As someone who has always been very self-sufficient, it was very hard for me to tell my colleagues at the office that I simply could not write patient notes all day long anymore. It was the first time that MS had impacted my work life. I did not like feeling "weak" in any way. But as is usually the case in these circumstances, I had made much more of the situation than anyone else did. Everyone in my office was very supportive and no one considered it a big deal that I would be using a dictation system all the time. Importantly, to my great delight, the strength in my arm was greatly improved after just two weeks of staying away from a pen.

# 13

# GETTING INVOLVED WITH THE MS COMMUNITY

This chapter comes toward the end of the book for good reason. Getting involved with groups or organizations that have anything to do with MS may not be something that immediately comes to mind when you are facing a new diagnosis of MS. In an earlier chapter, I mentioned that I had attended an educational fundraiser for MS a few years ago where I met a woman who had recently been diagnosed with MS. Our personalities definitely "clicked" that day, and we ultimately went on to become friends. However, there was one very big difference between the two of us at the fundraiser that day. While I had been diagnosed with MS four years earlier, it had only been a few months since she had been diagnosed. Her courage and willingness to get involved in the MS community so early on in her diagnosis astonished me. When I was only a few months into my diagnosis, I was still not comfortable saying the words *multiple sclerosis* out loud, never mind going to a fundraiser for MS.

Talking about "getting involved in the MS community" can sound as if you are going to be required to give of yourself or of your time in one way or another. Many of you may never feel sure about giving any more of yourselves when you are already working so hard to incorporate your health issues into the balance of your everyday life. Yet, one of the reasons for writing this chapter is to show you how getting involved can also be all about getting something back for yourself in return. There are countless different ways and degrees to which you can get involved in the MS community, and each setting has different benefits to offer. You may consider the possibility of meeting just a few others living with MS by joining a small support group. Or perhaps, you are thinking about taking an active role in one of the larger MS organizations.

## SUPPORT GROUPS AND SELF-HELP GROUPS

At first, the very thought of attending a support group meeting can be intimidating. You may have concerns about being asked to share too much personal information about yourself when you are not ready to do so yet. You may have the perception that everyone attending such a meeting tries to maintain an upbeat and positive attitude when you are not yet feeling positive. Others may worry that support groups are too "touchy–feely."

Remember that an MS support group is made up of individuals who have experienced many of the same emotions and situations that you have. After having talked to very sympathetic family members, friends, and physicians over the years, no one else understands the issues I am dealing with in the same way that another person with multiple sclerosis does. The first time you choose to walk in the door to attend a support group meeting, everyone else in that room remembers the way they felt when they walked in the door the first time too. No one there will ask for any information until you feel ready to share it.

Reasons to initially consider joining a support group may be the need to know that you are not alone in living with MS or in feeling the way you do. If you have not yet attended any sort of MS event, you may not know anyone else living with MS. It may be helpful to hear how others coped with the diagnosis when it was still new. You may find practical solutions for some of your own issues as you hear others describe how they handled similar challenges with home or work life. There may be a component of curiosity to know what types of disabilities others with MS have faced and how they have dealt with them. More than anything, you may benefit just from knowing that there is a truly understanding person who is listening to what you have to say.

I had the opportunity to take part in a group conversation that was very much like a support group when I attended a patient-oriented seminar about "Multiple Sclerosis and the Eye." The physician giving the lecture stated that the pain of optic neuritis usually resolves during the first few weeks or months after the initial diagnosis. Within seconds, many of the people in the audience who had previously had optic neuritis began whispering to each other. Throughout our whispers, we were all expressing concerns that we did not think the statement about resolution of eye pain after optic neuritis was entirely accurate. A surprising number of us still experienced eye pain with various activities including reading or computer work, or during times of extreme stress or fatigue.

After the seminar, many of us from the audience sat and chatted with each other for quite some time. We were amazed to hear each other describe such similar sensations and symptoms in our eyes. It validated for each of us that we "were not crazy" despite the fact that our eyes were supposed to be pain-free after the initial inflammation from our optic neuritis had resolved. We joked that we should have formed our impromptu support group much sooner.

Another benefit that we may not think about as we contemplate joining a support group is the great service we can provide to other people with MS simply by providing an empathetic and nonjudgmental ear. If you also have MS, then you *have* been there. You *do* know what other people in the group are talking about. The first time I was the one listening to the fear in the voice of a young woman who was newly diagnosed with MS, I felt a great sense of satisfaction as I saw the relief in her face after she shared some of her worries with me. She knew that I understood completely. All I had done to alleviate some of her anxiety was to listen. So if you think you may not have anything to offer to a support group, think again.

Multiple sclerosis support groups and self-help groups come in all different "shapes and sizes." When I scan my quarterly edition of *MS Connection*, a newsletter put out by the National Multiple Sclerosis Society (NMSS), I see support groups listed for those who are newly diagnosed, minimally disabled, Christian-oriented, primary progressive MS, men only, African Americans, and the list goes on. Of course, there are an equal number of support groups that are for all-comers with MS. There are many different organizations responsible for the creation of various support groups including the NMSS, the pharmaceutical companies who manufacture the disease-modifying drugs, and several Internet MS organizations. "Support groups" may have professional facilitators, while the "self-help groups" are frequently led by someone in the group with MS. If you are considering joining a support group, take some time to look into the various options in your area so that you may locate a group that will meet your current needs. (Please see the Resource Guide at the end of the book for a more complete list of organizations.)

## MULTIPLE SCLEROSIS ORGANIZATIONS

I am not sure exactly how long it took after my diagnosis before I decided to become a member of the NMSS, but I am certain that it was at least two years. There was something about becoming a member of a well-known, national organization that somehow made my diagnosis seem more "official." Because there is a check box on the registration form where it asks if you know anyone with multiple sclerosis, it seemed like a very formal process to report to such an organization that I am actually the one with MS. (Of course, you are not required to provide any of that information.)

Over the years, I have slowly increased my participation with the NMSS as I have become more comfortable in doing so. While I think it is wonderful that they exist to support research for MS and to provide a wealth of services to those living with MS, I initially wondered if there would be any personal, positive impact on my life by joining such an organization. Now that I have taken part in a variety of events sponsored by the NMSS during the past several years, I am certain that there have been tremendous benefits for me as an individual by belonging to such an organization. I feel this way despite never having received any formal services or assistance from the organization as of yet.

So what kind of benefits am I talking about? The first local NMSS-sponsored event I attended was a silent auction and dance. This is an annual event held in our city with a 1920s theme so that all of the attendees are encouraged to come dressed in costumes from that era. Initially, I was very sheepish about going. I had the usual concerns that many of us experience when we attend any event that involves wearing a costume. I felt slightly awkward in my rented 1920s dress, and I hoped that many others would also arrive in costume. However, my greater concern was whether or not I would end up telling many people at the event that I was there because I have MS. At that point, I had not been very open about my MS in public settings, in part because I never wanted to sense that anyone was feeling sorry for me.

The event turned out to be an incredible eye opener for me. The rooms were full of more young people than I had ever imagined would be there, and they had all come to have a good time. I realized that because MS affects many individuals who are in their twenties and thirties, a great deal of support is going to come from family and friends who are also in that age bracket. The attendees were not limited to the young, however. There was an incredibly diverse group of people of all ages and backgrounds, some with canes or scooters, and all with smiles on their faces.

The atmosphere that night was extremely festive and upbeat. When I did choose to tell others there about my MS, I felt completely supported, but I never felt anyone's pity. This came as a great relief to me. I was also surprised by how many "me too" responses I got when I revealed my own diagnosis. I left that evening feeling much better about living with multiple sclerosis. I had met many great people with MS. I had seen an outpouring of community support to combat the disease. I realized that I *would* be able to deal with MS over the years, just as so many others in that room had been doing. I truly felt more hopeful as I left the event that I had initially had so many concerns about attending.

The other NMSS-sponsored event that I have come to look forward to each year is our local chapter's annual walk. At the beginning, I also had some reservations about participating in this type of event. While I was interested in raising money to support MS research, I was not necessarily ready to be a cheerleader for the cause. Participating in the walk seemed like taking a big step. In addition to raising money, much of the concept surrounding the walk is to raise public awareness about MS. If I were to participate in the walk, then I thought I should feel ready to "go public" about my MS. The first year that I decided to attend the walk, there were not many people beyond my immediate family and close friends that knew I had MS. Of course, this notion of having to reveal my diagnosis to more people in order to participate in such events was something construed entirely in my own mind.

Just as I had come to realize with the 1920s-themed fundraiser, I soon recognized that I had placed far too much emphasis on the implications of participating in the annual walk. No one at the walk would be focusing on me as an individual person living with MS. Instead, the annual walk is a celebration and recognition of all of those whose lives have been affected by MS. I saw again that when such an organization gets together, it is not at all about doom and gloom. There was music and there were many happy faces. Yet, there was also an acknowledgment that we still need to make much greater strides in our understanding and treatment of MS. There was a genuine sense of commitment from everyone walking that day to support the researchers in their efforts to find better treatments and ultimately a cure for MS.

As I have continued to take part in various MS events over the years, I have found myself moving beyond my self-centered concerns about being a visible and active member in the MS community. As I have become more comfortable in being able to say, " I have multiple sclerosis," I have realized that I might actually have something to give back to others in the community. Approximately two years ago, the desire to give something back to others with MS began to take hold of me, and I decided to act on that feeling. Now, when I do take advantage of the opportunities to give something back, whether by talking to a support group or by being a patient advocate, the personal rewards are tremendous. Each time, I am touched by the lives of others who share part of their MS experience with me.

## What Can an MS Group Do for Me?

You have read about my personal experiences and about my perceptions of the benefits that may come from being involved in the MS community. (And, please keep in mind that I do not formally represent the NMSS. I have described some of their events through my own eyes.) But what can getting involved in the MS community do for you? As different as we all are, we will have many different reasons why we may or may not want to consider participation with any type of MS group or organization. Some of you may be like my friend who was attending a fundraiser within months of her diagnosis. From the initial time of her diagnosis, she has lived with an attitude of "taking on this disease" and doing whatever she can to stop it in its tracks. Others may be more like I was at the beginning with feelings of uncertainty about being ready to jump into anything.

Wherever you are in your personal journey in living with MS, it is helpful to be aware that such organizations and resources exist. While I have highlighted some of the fundraising events that an organization like the NMSS does, they also provide an incredible array of services to those with MS. Much of my discussion of difficult topics covered in other chapters came with the recommendation that you consider seeking professional advice or counseling on matters related to career, children, disability, or other health concerns. When you are trying to figure out how to locate such a professional, the MS organizations or support groups can assist you in finding the person you need. In addition and very important, the NMSS plays an incredible role in advocacy for all of us living with MS. When an important new medication for MS was withdrawn from the market, the NMSS was involved in the hearings that eventually led to the drug's availability again. When the government-regulated prescription drug coverage changed, the NMSS also made our voices heard.

A visit to the Web sites of the NMSS and the pharmaceutical-sponsored patient support groups will introduce you to the spectrum of services they can provide. These websites also include a listing of the many educational materials that are available to you.

## FINDING THE RIGHT FIT FOR YOU

Just because I encourage you to explore the benefits of becoming involved in the MS community, I clearly recognize that being part of an MS support group or organization in a public or social way will not be for everyone. Even if you prefer never to attend a meeting or social event sponsored by one of these groups, I would still suggest that you think about becoming a member "on paper" or on-line. Once you have registered through the mail or on-line, you will then receive the various publications distributed by these organizations.

I look forward to reading the magazines and literature that come from both the manufacturer of my MS medication as well as from the NMS Society. These publications address issues that are pertinent and practical for those of us living with MS. In these magazines, I have read about topics ranging from job discrimination or disability to dealing with depression or the heat. The publications also keep me updated on current research and any new drugs that may be forthcoming. Even if I were never talking to anyone else with MS, the magazines and Web sites would allow me to feel connected with the MS community. After reading one of the publications, I am reminded that I am not the only one in the world living with MS. I close the magazines feeling better informed about what is going on in the MS world.

Give yourself time to find the setting that is right for you. Whether you choose to quietly read an MS magazine in the privacy of your own home, to join a small support group, or to participate in every major MS event that comes your way, I encourage you to find some way to allow the "MS community" into your life. Having that feeling of connectedness to others with MS can provide an ongoing source of strength and reassurance.

# 14

## FINDING BALANCE

A year after my diagnosis, I was casually talking with a physician friend at work about the fact that my husband and I were contemplating a move to another part of the country. This would be a major move for us as my husband had thus far lived all of his thirty-four years in the same state. His parents and siblings all lived within a short drive from us. Yet, I really longed for a warmer climate, a less stressful job, and a slightly different way of life. My friend's response to me was, "You only go through this life once. Life is not a dress rehearsal. You need to get it right the first time."

Six years later, I continue to reflect on those words as I strive to find a healthy balance in my life. While none of us with MS would choose to have it, I suspect that many of us eventually reach a point where we can admit that having been diagnosed with MS caused us to think about what is really important in life. How do we make the most of today if there is some uncertainty about our health in the future? What do we value most and what are our highest priorities in our homes, our work, and our social lives? Some have told me that a diagnosis of MS sent them down a spiritual or religious path not previously explored. Although it would be wonderful if we had previously addressed all of these questions, sometimes it takes such a diagnosis to stop us in the tracks of our busy lives and encourage us to evaluate what we are doing and where we are headed.

As I started to write this chapter, I joked with my husband and friends that I had hoped I would have found balance in my life by the time I was ready to write such a chapter. As they watch me run from work to volunteering at school to coaching soccer while being a mom and trying to write a book in my "free time," they wonder how I could write a chapter about finding balance with any wisdom to share. While I freely admit that I have some distance to go before I achieve what may be the ideal balance, I know that I have already contemplated some difficult questions that ultimately led to beneficial changes for my physical and mental health in living with MS.

## WHAT IS IT THAT WE ARE BALANCING?

Since we are going to be managing our MS for a lifetime, we need to find a healthy balance in our lives that falls somewhere in between throwing in the towel because we have a chronic illness and being superwoman or superman to prove that we can do anything we want to do. Within the first few days of my diagnosis, I definitely had brief passing thoughts of "Well, at least now I have a really good reason not to keep working so hard. People with MS don't have to keep a crazy schedule like mine." In the beginning, I believe it is a normal reaction to consider a diagnosis of MS to be a reason to take a back seat to life's responsibilities and challenges. We are feeling emotionally overwhelmed, and we may be dealing with a number of different physical symptoms. Applying for disability from our job may sound like a welcome relief. Allowing our partner or roommate to take care of all the household responsibilities may not sound so bad.

At the time of diagnosis, a break from work, school, or other responsibilities for a brief period of time may be exactly what we need. Fortunately, within a few weeks or months, many of us will find ourselves in a position where we are physically and mentally capable of resuming many of our previous activities and responsibilities. Most of us will move beyond that initial desire to escape from work or school as we realize that withdrawing from many of our usual activities would likely leave us feeling empty and unfulfilled.

At the other end of the spectrum are those who are sometimes referred to as "workaholics" and cannot imagine slowing down. This may be a businessperson who works long, hard hours each week to achieve success in a career. Or, it may be a college student getting straight As while participating in countless extra-curricular activities. These individuals may be tempted to jump right back into life's hectic pace as soon as they are feeling well enough. There may be the desire to say, "Hey, look at all that I am doing. MS is not going to slow me down one little bit." While I would never discourage any of us from pursing goals or accomplishing great tasks, I would always encourage us to do so in a manner that feels emotionally and physically healthy.

In striving for a healthy balance between doing too little and doing too much, there may be a need to look carefully at your current situation. Beyond examining the details of daily living, such as workspace configurations or finding time to nap, striving for balance in your life means looking at the big picture. It means asking yourself what you value most and what your priorities are. These are sometimes hard questions to ask. Is my current job well suited for me? Is my school load too much? Am I involved in activities that I enjoy? How is my family life?

Although I was not consciously asking myself these particular questions after my diagnosis, I definitely began to think about what I valued most in life. How did I feel about working five long days each week while my children were with a caretaker? What did I see as my long-term career goals? If I could not be assured of good physical health several years down the road, was I currently doing the things that I enjoyed that required good physical health? As I thought about such issues, my children's play dates, school parties, and soccer games began to take on greater importance. The pace of my life started to appear quite hectic from the outside looking in, so I slowly began the process of simplifying certain aspects.

Of course, these are very personal examples of questions I asked myself. Your questions will be as unique as you are. It is important to realize that just because we ask questions of ourselves as we strive for balance in our lives, it does not mean that the changes we may want to make will be readily available options. Perhaps you will conclude that cutting back on the number of hours you put in at work each week would be best for your health, home, or family life. Yet, your workplace may not currently have an option for reduced hours. Or, working fewer hours may result in financial hardship that would not be acceptable. Regardless of initial obstacles you may encounter, I encourage you to explore your options.

## WILL TOO MUCH STRESS WORSEN MY MS?

As I talk about setting priorities and encourage you to "take time to smell the flowers," there is the implication that many of our lives are busy and stressful. While I cannot assume that every reader of this book would say that his life is stressful, I do know from talking to hundreds of patients every month that many people living in our country today find life to be taking place at a fairly rapid pace. This does not mean that we are not enjoying the things we do. However, it means that an element of stress sneaks in at least once in a while for most of us.

If we are enjoying the jobs and activities we do and we are still capable of doing them, is there any reason to talk about simplifying things? If we experience an element of stress on a regular basis from all that we do, could this have a negative long-term effect on the course of our MS? While I discussed this question in an earlier chapter that referred specifically to job stress, life stressors can be of many different forms. Stress many come from running a busy household, from balancing the checkbook every week, or from caring for an older parent. The scientific studies that have tried to answer the question about the impact of stress on multiple sclerosis have looked at the effect of major life stressors occurring in the lives of those living with MS. These studies evaluated the effects of stressors such as loss of a loved one, a severe illness, or the loss of a job. Not surprisingly, such dramatic life events were associated with an increase in MS relapses.[1] However, it is much more difficult to research the impact of living a hectic life where there is a persistent, low to moderate level of stress taking place each day.

Many physicians and nonphysicians have drawn their own similar conclusions about daily stress and its potential negative impact on health. I certainly recognize that many of my patients with illnesses such as high blood pressure or diabetes tend to have better control of their disease process when they feel less stressed. It is not uncommon for me to see a patient whose blood pressure has been difficult to control to suddenly have a great improvement in blood pressure when he or she switches to a less stressful job or retires. In living with MS, I think it is plausible that high levels of everyday stress may play a role in the number of exacerbations we have over the years. Even if there is no proven relationship between everyday stress and actual exacerbations, stress certainly has the potential to play a role in the level of fatigue we experience and in our desire and ability to make our health a priority.

As I consider the potential impact of daily stress on our lives, I again emphasize the importance of finding a healthy balance. If we chose to take a backseat to all of life's activities that might cause us some degree of stress, we would likely suffer from lack of mental stimulation and social interaction. I know I have already said many times in this book that I believe that it is so very important that we continue to be active participants in our homes, communities, and workplaces. Yet, only we can decide as individuals where that healthy balance lies.

## REJUVENATING

Several months ago, I was attending an educational seminar on multiple sclerosis with a girlfriend who also has MS. During one of the breaks, she asked me if I had gone for my massage yet that month. I laughed. I told her that sounded lovely, but I simply did not have time to go and get a massage on any regular basis. She told me that she tried to keep up with a massage almost every month. Not only did having a massage serve as a big stress reliever for her, but it made her feel physically better in terms of her MS.

Going for a regular massage may seem like quite an indulgence. It can also come with a significant price tag. (Occasionally, therapeutic massage will be covered by health insurance.) Yet, my friend's question made me realize how important it is to make the time for the activities that we find to be relaxing and rejuvenating. This may be as simple as a thirty-minute nap every day. Or, perhaps, you may spend thirty minutes of each day reading a good book, watching a favorite show, or listening to music. Of course, taking a few minutes each day to relax and rejuvenate is important for everyone in our busy society. Yet, I am also convinced that my chronic arm and leg numbness is so much better on the days when I build in time for a few minutes of rest and relaxation.

## KEEP STRIVING FOR THE BALANCE

As a result of being diagnosed with MS, I took a closer look at my life and evaluated what was most important to me. I think I am more likely to look back some day and feel good about some of the hard decisions I have made to set priorities and focus on my values. I decided to slow down the crazy rollercoaster ride that was becoming my very hectic life. Each day, I still look for ways to put the brakes on a little bit more because I know that I have not quite achieved the balance that I would like to have.

What is important to you in your life? How are you feeling physically, mentally, and emotionally? Are there changes you should consider making because of physical or emotional issues that have surfaced as a result of your MS? Where can you do some fine-tuning to allow your priorities to surface? Asking these questions and attempting to put the solutions into place is what finding balance is all about. While the scales may always feel a little lopsided, as long as we remain mindful of looking for balance in our lives, we are likely to feel much better than if we had never given it any thought.

# CONCLUSION

Multiple sclerosis is the name that has been given to a process that causes damage to the protective coating around the nerves in the central nervous system. "Multiple sclerosis" is certainly not my personal name, and having multiple sclerosis does not define who I am. In the beginning, however, I did sometimes feel as if "multiple sclerosis" was a new name that I had been given. I was very afraid that the illness would somehow define me as a person. I was sure that my life as I knew it would never be the same again.

In actuality, living my life with MS has not been exactly the same as it was before my diagnosis, but not because of any of the reasons I had feared so intensely. It is my hope that the thoughts and stories shared in this book have shown you that a diagnosis of MS is not going to rob you of the good things in life. There are going to be challenges along the way. Some days, or even weeks, will be more frustrating than others. There may be modifications that you need to make in the ways you accomplish certain tasks or in the activities that you choose to do. Yet overall, your life can march forward in many of the same ways as you had always planned.

I continue to work as a physician, but I work three days each week instead of five. I dictate my patient notes more often than my colleagues do in order to avoid writing with a numb right arm. I still coach soccer, but I rush to get back inside to an air-conditioned environment after coaching on a hot day. There are definitely times when I choose to pass on the opportunity to participate in an activity because I know it will be too much for me. (Trying to jog with my girlfriends is no longer worth the resulting heat exhaustion and heavy leg.) Yet, in passing on one particular activity, I have frequently discovered a new interest that I may not have otherwise explored.

Friends tell me that I have a "glass half-full" approach in living my life with MS. It took a long time for that glass to look half-full to me instead of half-empty. If it has been a short time since your diagnosis, the passage of time alone will make a tremendous difference in how you view your own situation. Your outlook is likely to be greatly improved six or twelve months from now.

We live in an era of highly effective treatments to decrease the frequency of exacerbations in relapsing–remitting MS. The majority of us diagnosed with RRMS in the past ten to fifteen years remain active participants in our families, workplace, and communities. The longer you live with and learn to manage your MS, the more you will come to know the truth in that statement.

I would never go so far as to say that I am glad for having been diagnosed with MS. I would much rather have more energy and less numbness, tingling and dizziness. It would be wonderful if I did not have to stick myself with a needle on a regular basis. (And, I do really miss being able to go on the spinning rides with my children!) However, I do believe that being diagnosed with MS eventually led me to think critically about what matters most to me in life. I would like to think that I would have made those same discoveries without ever having been diagnosed with MS. That I will never know.

The chapters in this book discussed the various symptoms, challenges, and situations that may arise in living with MS. While the solutions will be different for each of you, I hope you have come to see that you are not alone in your experience of these situations or in the emotions that may accompany them. Not only do we live in an era of highly effective medications for MS, but we also live in a time with countless different professionals and resources to help us navigate through the challenges that come our way. Do not hesitate to seek them out.

## HOPE

The word *hope* is commonly used in a number of slogans for multiple sclerosis organizations and events. It was very important to me that the word hope appeared somewhere on the cover of this book. More than anything, it was my intention in writing this book that you would be able to turn the last page believing that there is every reason to maintain hope for the future.

# Appendix: The Facts about MS

This appendix presents basic facts about multiple sclerosis. It is an overview for someone without a medical background. Several other books and resources, listed in the "Resources" section, provide a more detailed explanation of the medical aspects of multiple sclerosis.

## What Is Multiple Sclerosis (MS)?

Multiple sclerosis is a disease that damages the nerves in the brain and spinal cord. The brain and spinal cord make up the central nervous system, which receives sensory input from the nerves and signals the body to take action. While the exact cause is not known, MS is considered to be an *autoimmune* disease because the body's own immune system is involved in the attack on the nervous system. *Myelin* is the specific component of the nervous system that comes under attack in MS.

Myelin is the material that forms a protective sheath around the nerve fibers. *Axon* is the medical term for these nerve fibers. In multiple sclerosis, a process called *demyelination* occurs as the myelin is attacked and the axons lose their protective coating. Without myelin, nerve cells lose their ability to transmit electrical signals effectively. Such attacks on myelin play a role in the relapses and the clinical symptoms that people with MS experience. Over time, in addition to damaging myelin, MS can cause axons to be severed—and it is this process that may be responsible for some of the permanent disability of MS.

The word "multiple" in MS comes from the fact that multiple different areas of the brain and spinal cord may be affected. "Sclerosis" is a term that refers to the scar tissue that can form in the area of damaged nerves. Multiple sclerosis is a heterogeneous disease, which means that individual patients may have very different symptoms from each other and that individual patients will respond differently to the various medications.

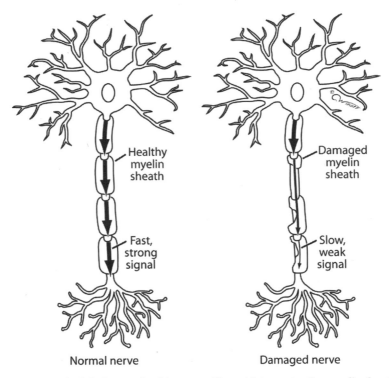

The figure on the left shows a healthy nerve fiber with its protective myelin sheath. On the right is a myelin sheath damaged by the disease process in multiple sclerosis. *Illustration by Christopher Wikoff, CMI, 2007.*

## WHAT CAUSES MS?

The answer to this question remains under intensive investigation. Many researchers believe that some type of environmental trigger turns on the autoimmune response, allowing the body's immune system to inappropriately attack its own nervous system. In addition to environmental factors, genes may play a role. Studies have shown that, while there is not a single gene allowing multiple sclerosis to occur, certain specific gene patterns are found in people with MS, suggesting a genetic predisposition to the disease. As for the actual environmental cause that serves as the trigger in those with a genetic predisposition, there have been many theories about different types of viruses or bacteria that may turn on the autoimmune attack. However, thus far, nothing definitive has been proven.

Because multiple sclerosis is more common in higher latitudes where there is less sun exposure, research studies have examined the potential role of vitamin D deficiency in MS. (Sunlight is a major source of vitamin D.) While people who have higher blood levels of vitamin D seem to be diagnosed with MS less often than are those with lower levels, a definite cause and effect is unproven. Immune cells do have receptors for vitamin D, so it is certainly possible that vitamin D plays a protective role for individuals who are at risk for MS.

Although precise triggers for the onset of disease are unknown, scientists do know quite a bit about what goes wrong with the immune system at the cellular level in multiple sclerosis. A group of cells known as *T cells* play a very important role in the everyday functioning of a healthy immune system, as they help to attack and eradicate viruses and bacteria that the body may encounter. The only time T cells should enter the brain and cross through what is known as the *blood-brain barrier* is when there is infection in the brain itself.

In multiple sclerosis, however, these T cells have been improperly activated to cross the blood-brain barrier even when no infection is present. Once within the brain, the T cells inappropriately attack the myelin coating on the nerve fibers. What takes place in this attack is a complex process on the cellular level. The majority of current treatments for relapsing–remitting MS work by preventing or altering this attack on myelin by the T cells. The various MS medications work at different steps in the process.

## Who Gets MS?

Multiple sclerosis is approximately two to three times more common in women than in men. While multiple sclerosis can strike anyone, it is most common among white populations. When specific ancestries are examined, people of Northern European descent appear to have the highest rate of MS. In the United States, African Americans, Native Americans, Hispanic Americans, and Asian Americans develop MS, although not as commonly as the Caucasian population does. Relapsing–remitting MS, which is the most common type of MS, generally begins when people are in their twenties or thirties. MS can occur in childhood, but it is rarely seen before age 10.

## Types of Multiple Sclerosis

### Relapsing–Remitting Multiple Sclerosis (RRMS)

Relapsing–remitting multiple sclerosis is the most common type of multiple sclerosis, affecting approximately 85 percent of patients at the *onset* of the disease. At any give time, 50 to 55 percent of the entire MS population is considered to have RRMS.

RRMS is characterized by discrete episodes of new neurological symptoms that are thought to occur because of a new occurrence of demyelination somewhere in the brain or spinal cord. An episode of a specific set of new symptoms is referred to as a *relapse* or an *exacerbation*. Examples of symptoms signaling a relapse include optic neuritis with visual loss in one eye, sudden weakness in a limb, double vision, dizziness or vertigo, or new sensory changes such as persistent numbness and tingling.

Relapses are usually followed by a period of recovery when most or all of the neurological symptoms resolve. This period of recovery is referred to as *remission.*

Over time, the recovery periods tend to be less complete in terms of a total return to the person's baseline neurological function before the relapse. Therefore, some degree of disability is usually accumulated by most people over the years. The majority of people diagnosed with RRMS, however, do not end up severely disabled. Recent studies also suggest that currently prescribed disease-modifying drugs not only prevent relapses but may also slow progression of the disease.[1] Therefore, there is good reason to believe that, now and in the future, long-term disabilities in people with MS will be less common and less debilitating than they were for people with the disease twenty-five years ago.

### Secondary Progressive Multiple Sclerosis

Secondary progressive multiple sclerosis was the eventual course for almost half of the people living with RRMS prior to the age of disease-modifying drugs. With this type of MS, after five to ten years of relapses and remissions, there comes a gradual worsening of neurological symptoms and function. Some people may still have periods of defined relapses during the secondary phase, but a slow functional decline still occurs, even without identifiable relapses. This decline is thought to be due in part to damage to the axons and resulting brain atrophy. At any given time, approximately 40 percent of people with MS have secondary progressive multiple sclerosis.

Whether the disease-modifying drugs will change the percentage of people who transition from relapsing–remitting MS to secondary progressive MS is not yet clear. With a disease like RRMS, it takes at least ten years to see such benefits after the introduction of new medications. As mentioned above, an observational study of RRMS patients concluded that the interferon drugs and glatirimer acetate slow the rate of disability progression when compared to the rate of disability progression in people who had never had the opportunity for medication.[1] While not a clinical trial, these results provide hope that these medications will have a long-term benefit.

### Primary Progressive Multiple Sclerosis

Primary progressive multiple sclerosis is characterized by a slow but continuous worsening of neurological symptoms or function from the very start of the disease. There are no clearly identifiable relapses in this form of the disease, although some people with PPMS can identify periods of stabilization, or "plateaus."

Primary progressive MS is a less common form of the disease, affecting approximately 10 percent of those living with MS. It tends to affect people who are older and is seen equally in women and men.

### Progressive Relapsing Multiple Sclerosis

This is the least common form of MS and is not always identified as a separate type of multiple sclerosis. As in primary progressive MS, with PRMS there is a continuous worsening of neurological function from the onset. However, people with this form of MS also have clearly identifiable relapses.

## Symptoms of Multiple Sclerosis

Because the central nervous system plays a critical role in the functioning of all five senses, all muscle groups, and some organs and because MS affects the central nervous system, many different symptoms can potentially occur as a result of multiple sclerosis. The list below is not meant to be comprehensive. It includes some of the more common symptoms and can appear frightening to anyone who has been newly diagnosed with multiple sclerosis. The majority of people with relapsing–remitting MS will experience a minority of these symptoms.

Symptoms in MS may also come and go. Major new symptoms can show up in the form of a relapse, and, in addition, chronic symptoms may be more strongly noticed or experienced on some days than others. These changes and their unpredictability are part of the disease. One example is that a person may have a particular area of the body that sometimes becomes numb, but it may not be numb all the time or to the same degree. Another example is that people who have been left with difficulty walking after a relapse may have some days when they walk better than other days.

## Possible Symptoms

| | |
|---|---|
| Fatigue | Balance problems / unsteadiness |
| Bladder dysfunction | Visual problems |
| Pain | Dizziness |
| Cognitive dysfunction (memory or reasoning) | Sexual dysfunction |
| Numbness/tingling | Spasticity / muscle tightness |
| Clumsiness | Weakness |
| Slurred speech | Depression |
| Gait disorders | |

## Treatment of Multiple Sclerosis

Treatment of MS can refer to three different aspects of disease management: (1) treatment to decrease the frequency of relapses, with the goal of decreasing or delaying long-term disability; (2) treatment to speed recovery from a relapse; or (3) treatment to control some of the longer-term symptoms that may persist after an exacerbation.

### Medications to Decrease Relapses

The medications used to decrease relapse frequency are commonly referred to as "disease-modifying drugs." As stated in Chapter 4, these medications are referred to this way because they do not actually cure multiple sclerosis, but they change the course of the illness (modify it) by decreasing the frequency of relapses and the emergence of new lesions as seen on an MRI. The four drugs

most commonly used for a new diagnosis of MS are Avonex, Betaseron, Copaxone, and Rebif. Novantrone and Tysabri are two other disease-modifying drugs
that are usually reserved for relapsing–remitting MS that is not responding well
to initial therapy or for secondary progressive MS.

The initiation of a disease-modifying medication is strongly recommended
after a diagnosis of multiple sclerosis has been confirmed. Delaying treatment
by just a few years after diagnosis can make it more difficult to control future
disease. In addition, there are now scientific data showing that treatment immediately after a first attack of a syndrome that is common in MS, such as optic
neuritis, will delay the onset to a definite diagnosis of MS.[2–4] Therefore, the
overwhelming message from scientists and neurologists is to initiate therapy as
early as possible.

Choosing which of the disease-modifying drugs to initiate is a decision usually made by a patient's neurologist, with strong consideration given to patient
preferences. Several recent studies have shown that the interferon drugs Rebif
and Betaseron are similarly effective when compared to Copaxone. Frequency
of dosing, method of administration (subcutaneous versus intramuscular), and
potential side effects may all play a role in the choice of initial therapy. Because
drug studies are always ongoing in MS research, results from a newly reported
study can also influence drug selection made by the neurologist.

What follows is a brief description of the current disease-modifying drugs,
including how they are administered and their potential side effects. It is extremely important to realize, in reviewing a list of potential side effects, that
the majority of patients do not experience these side effects. In addition, some
side effects, such as flu-like symptoms from the interferon drugs, may decrease
over time. The neurologist and the patient must work together to manage any
side effects that may emerge so the patient can continue to take the drug on
a long-term basis (this is called "patient compliance with drug treatment"). For
Web site addresses and support line telephone numbers for each medication,
please refer to Chapter 4.

Betaseron, or interferon beta-1b, was approved for relapsing forms of MS
in 1993 and is administered by subcutaneous injection every other day. It has
been shown to decrease the number and frequency of relapses as well as to
slow the progression of disease. Common side effects include flu-like symptoms
(fatigue, muscle aches, chills) and injection site reactions (redness, pain, or swelling). More serious but less common side effects include major depression, liver
problems, decrease in white blood cell counts, and injection site necrosis. (*Necrosis* refers to the breakdown of the skin and underlying fat where the injection was given.) Allergic reactions such as hives, rash, or itching have also been
reported. Life-threatening allergic reactions are rare. Betaseron should not be
taken during pregnancy or while breastfeeding.

Avonex, or interferon beta-1a, was approved for relapsing forms of MS in
1996 and is administered by intramuscular injection once weekly. It has been
shown to decrease the number and frequency of relapses as well as to slow
the progression of disease. A common side effect is flu-like symptoms (fatigue,

muscle aches, chills). More serious but less common side effects include major depression, liver problems, and decrease in blood cell count (both white cells and platelets). Allergic reactions such as hives, rash, or itching have also been reported. Life-threatening allergic reactions are rare. Avonex should not be taken during pregnancy or while breastfeeding.

Rebif, or interferon beta-1a, was approved for relapsing forms of MS in 2002 and is administered by subcutaneous injection three times each week. It has been shown to decrease the number and frequency of relapses as well as to slow the progression of disease. Common side effects include flu-like symptoms (fatigue, muscle aches, chills) and injection site reactions (redness, pain, or swelling). More serious but less common side effects include major depression, liver problems, decrease in white blood cell counts, and injection site necrosis. Allergic reactions such as hives, rash, or itching have also been reported. Life-threatening allergic reactions are rare. Rebif should not be taken during pregnancy or while breastfeeding.

Patients on Betaseron, Avonex, or Rebif should undergo regularly scheduled laboratory monitoring for blood cell counts and liver function.

Copaxone, or glatirimer acetate, was approved for relapsing forms of MS in 1996 and is administered daily by subcutaneous injection. It has been shown to decrease the number and frequency of relapses as well as to slow the progression of disease. The most common side effect is injection site reaction (redness, pain, or swelling). With prolonged use of Copaxone, some patients may experience lipoatrophy, or breakdown of the fatty layer underlying the skin. Flu-like symptoms are not experienced with Copaxone. A more serious but less common side effect is an immediate postinjection reaction that can include shortness of breath, heart palpitations, flushing, and anxiety. If this reaction occurs, it usually resolves on its own within several minutes and does not usually require medical intervention. Copaxone is the only MS-approved drug with a "category B" pregnancy rating, which means that it appears to be safe in pregnant laboratory animals receiving the drug, but it has not been tested in pregnant women.

Tysabri, or nataluzimab, was approved for relapsing forms of MS in 2006. Tysabri is an antibody that prevents T cells from gaining access to the brain and has been proven to be very effective in reducing relapses and slowing the progression of disability. It is administered as a once monthly infusion through a vein. Because Tysabri may very rarely cause a life-threatening infection of the brain called "progressive multifocal leukoencephalopathy" (PML), it is usually given only to people who have not had a good response to or cannot tolerate the interferon drugs or Copaxone. Patients taking Tysabri are required to enroll in a safety monitoring program in attempt to detect any signs of PML. Less serious effects of Tysabri can include headache, urinary tract and respiratory infections, fatigue, joint pain, and rash. Tysabri should not be taking during pregnancy or while nursing.

Novantrone, or mitoxantrone, was approved in 2000 for worsening relapsing–remitting MS, secondary progressive MS, and progressive relapsing MS. It has been shown to slow and reduce the progression of disability in people whose symptoms are worsening. It is not approved for primary progressive MS. Novantrone is administered as an infusion through a vein every 3 months. Because of the potential for damage to the heart, careful monitoring of heart function is performed throughout the entire time that a person is on the medication. There is also a limit of total dose that can be given because of potential heart damage.

### Treatment of Relapses

Relapses are sometimes treated with medications called corticosteroids, which are known to have an anti-inflammatory effect. Prednisone, methylprednisolone, and dexamethasone are examples of corticosteroids. In some studies, these medications have been shown to shorten the duration of the relapse. However, corticosteroids do not change the long-term outcome of the relapse in terms of persistence of symptoms or the chances of having another relapse.

### Treatment of Specific MS Symptoms

Last, the various symptoms of MS are treated with medications directed at whatever the specific problem may be. As an example, problems with bladder control can be treated with medications that are used for an overactive bladder. Numbness and tingling that becomes uncomfortable can be treated with medications aimed at decreasing the perception of those sensations. Muscle tightness or spasticity can be treated with muscle relaxants. There are targeted treatment options for each of the symptoms listed above, under "Possible Symptoms"; the treatment options may consist of medication, physical or occupational therapy, or both. Many therapies can be explored to help with a given symptom, so it is of utmost importance to share those symptoms with the treating physician.

### Future Medications

This is an exciting time in MS research. An explosion of studies are under way to investigate new medications for relapsing forms of MS. Within three to five years of this publication, a number of new drugs will likely come to market in the form of oral, injectable, and intravenous medications.

# RESOURCES

The following lists are not meant to be inclusive of all possible MS groups and organizations. The list includes organizations or sites with which the author has had an opportunity to interact and has found to be helpful.

## MULTIPLE SCLEROSIS ORGANIZATIONS/WEB SITES

**Consortium of Multiple Sclerosis Services.** A site for the professional treating and researching MS. For the patient, a resource for current research, journal articles, and lectures.
www.mscare.org

**MSWorld.** A partner with the NMSS, this site focuses on individual experiences with MS. Provides a chat room and message board.
www.msworld.org

**Multiple Sclerosis International Federation.** An international site that links people together from all over the world living with MS. Up-to-date, thorough, and very informative.
www.msif.org

**National Multiple Sclerosis Society (NMSS)**
733 Third Avenue, 3rd Floor, New York, NY 10017
1-800-FIGHT-MS (1-800-344-4867)
www.nationalmssociety.org
email: info@nmss.org

**Rocky Mountain MS Center.** A comprehensive resource for complementary and alternative medical treatments for MS.
www.ms-cam.org

## Pharmaceutical Company–Sponsored Web Sites

**Berlex Labs, Inc.**
www.betaseron.com or www.mspathways.com
1-800-788-1467

**Biogen Idec**
www.avonex.com or www.msactivesource.com
1-800-456-2255

**Biogen Idec & Elan Pharmaceuticals**
www.tysabri.com
1-800-456-2255

**Serono, Inc.**
www.rebif.com or www.mslifelines.com or www.novantrone.com
1-877-447-3243

**TEVA Neurosciences, Inc.**
www.copaxone.com or www.sharedsolutions.com or www.mswatch.com
1-800-877-8100

## Disability Resources

**ABLEDATA.** Information about assistive technology & rehabilitation equipment. 8630 Fenton Street, Suite 390, Silver Spring, MD 20910, 1-800-227-0216
www.abledata.com

**ADA Home Page (Americans with Disabilities Act)**
www.usdoj.gov/crt/ada

**Descriptive Video Services.** Programs and movie services for those with impaired vision. 125 Western Avenue, WGBH, Boston, MA 02134, 1-800-333-1203
www.wgbh.org/dvs/
email: access@wgbh.org

**Disabled Online.** Extensive resources provided and a variety of topics covered.
www.disabledonline.com

## EMPLOYMENT AND DISABILITY

**Equal Employment Opportunity Commission**
www.eeoc.gov/types/ada

**Social Security Administration**
1-800-772-1213
www.ssa.gov/disability
For the "Blue Book" with exact requirements for Social Security Disability
Insurance Benefits: www.ssa.gov/disability/professionals/blue book

## GENERAL WELLNESS SITES

**Centers for Disease Control and Prevention—Physical Fitness Site**
www.cdc.gov/nccdphp/dnpa/physical/index.htm

**U.S. Department of Agriculture Food and Nutrition Information Center**
www.nal.usda.gov/fnic (Complete dietary resource)
www.mypyramid.gov (Develop a personal eating plan)

## OTHER MULTIPLE SCLEROSIS BOOKS IN PRINT

*Blindsided—Lifting a Life above Illness: A Reluctant Memoir.* By Richard Cohen.
Harper Paperbacks.
*Complementary and Alternative Medicine and Multiple Sclerosis,* 2nd Edition. By
Allen C. Bowling, MD, PhD. Demos Medical Publishing.
*Curing MS: How Science Is Solving the Mysteries of Multiple Sclerosis.* By Howard L. Weiner, MD. Three Rivers Press.
*Exercises for Multiple Sclerosis: A Safe and Effective Program to Fight Fatigue, Build
Strength, and Improve Balance.* By Brad Hamler. Hatherleigh Publishers.
*Living beyond Multiple Sclerosis: A Woman's Guide.* By Judith Lynn Nichols.
Hunter House.
*Managing the Symptoms of Multiple Sclerosis,* 5th Edition. By Randall Schapiro.
Demos Medical Publishing.
*Multiple Sclerosis: A Guide for Families.* By Rosalind Kalb, PhD. Demos Medical
Publishing.
*Multiple Sclerosis: A Self-Care Guide to Wellness,* 2nd Edition. By Nancy J. Holland and June Halper. Demos Medical Publishing.
*Multiple Sclerosis: Understanding the Cognitive Changes.* By Nicholas LaRocca,
PhD, and Rosalind Kalb, PhD. Demos Medical Publishing.
*Multiple Sclerosis Q&A: Reassuring Answers to Frequently Asked Questions.* By
Beth Ann Hill. Avery Publishing.

*The MS Workbook: Living Fully with Multiple Sclerosis.* By George Kraft, MD, Dawn M. Ehde, PhD, Kurt L. Johnson, PhD, and Robert T. Fraser. New Harbinger Publications.

*Speedbumps: Flooring It through Hollywood.* By Teri Garr. Plume Publishing.

*When Walking Fails.* By Lisa L. Iezzoni. University of California Press.

# REFERENCES

## CHAPTER 2

1. Kubler-Ross, E. *On Death and Dying*. New York: Macmillan, 1969.

## CHAPTER 6

1. Mohr, D.C., et al. 2004. Association between stressful life events and exacerbation in multiple sclerosis: A meta-analysis. *British Medical Journal* 328: 731–735.

## CHAPTER 7

1. Confavreux, C., et al. 1998. Rate of pregnancy-related relapse in multiple sclerosis. *The New England Journal of Medicine* 339: 285–291.

2. Vukusic, S., and Confavreux, C. 2006. Pregnancy and multiple sclerosis: The children of PRIMS *Clinical Neurology and Neurosurgery* 108: 266–270.

## CHAPTER 8

1. Oken, B.S., et al. 2004. Randomized controlled trial of yoga and exercise in multiple sclerosis. *Neurology* 62: 2058–2064.

2. Romberg, A., et al. 2004. Effects of a 6-month exercise program on patients with multiple sclerosis. *Neurology* 63: 2034–2038.

3. Munger, K.L., et al. 2006. Serum 25-hydroxyvitamin D levels and risk of multiple sclerosis. *JAMA* 296: 2832–2838.

4. Hayes, C.E., et al. 2003. The immunological functions of the vitamin D endocrine system. *Cellular and Molecular Biology* 49: 277–300.

5. Nordvik, I., et al. 2001. Effect of dietary advice and n-3 supplementation in newly diagnosed MS patients. *Acta Neurologica Scandinavia* 102: 143–149.

6. Weinstock-Guttman, B., et al. 2005. Low fat dietary intervention with omega-3 fatty acid supplementation in multiple sclerosis patients. *Prostaglandins, Leukotrienes and Essential Fatty Acids* 73: 397–404.

# CHAPTER 9

1. Stratmoen, J. 2006. On the job with fatigue and cognitive issues. *Inside MS* Feb–Mar: 24–29.

# CHAPTER 10

1. Patten, S.B., et al. 2003. Major depression in multiple sclerosis: A population-based perspective. *Neurology* 61: 1524–1527.

2. Bakshi, R., et al. 2000. Brain MRI lesions and atrophy are related to depression in multiple sclerosis. *Neuroreport* 11: 1153–1158.

3. Feinstein, A., et al. 2004. Structural brain lesions in multiple sclerosis patients with major depression. *Neurology* 62: 586–590.

4. Jacobs, L.D., et al. 2000. Intramuscular interferon beta-1a therapy initiated during a first demyelinating event in multiple sclerosis. *New England Journal of Medicine* 343: 898–904.

5. Patten, S.B., et al. 2002. Interferon beta-1a and depression in secondary progressive MS: Data from the SPECTRIMS trial. *Neurology* 59: 744–746.

6. Patten, S.B., et al. 2000. Biopsychosocial correlates of lifetime major depression in a multiple sclerosis population. *Multiple Sclerosis* 6: 115–120.

# CHAPTER 12

1. Bain, L.J., and Schapiro, R.T. 2007. *Managing MS through Rehabilitation.* National Multiple Sclerosis Library, Brochures.

# CHAPTER 14

1. Mohr, D.C., et al. 2004. Association between stressful life events and exacerbation in multiple sclerosis: A meta-analysis. *British Medical Journal* 328: 731–735.

# APPENDIX

1. Brown, M.G., et al. 2007. How effective are disease-modifying drugs in delaying progression in relapsing-onset MS? *Neurology* 69: 1498–1507.

2. Kappos, L., et al. 2007. A 3-year follow-up analysis of the BENEFIT study. *Lancet* 370: 389–397.

3. Comi, G., et al. 2001. Effect of early interferon treatment on conversion to definite MS: A randomised study. *Lancet* 357: 1576–1582.

4. Jacobs, L.D., et al. 2000. Intramuscular interferon beta-1a therapy initiated during a first demyelinating event in multiple sclerosis. *New England Journal of Medicine* 343: 898–904.

# INDEX

## About the Author

KYM ORSETTI FURNEY, M.D., is in private practice at Mecklenberg Medical Group of Carolinas Healthcare System in Charlotte, North Carolina. She is also Adjunct Associate Clinical Professor at the University of North Carolina School of Medicine. Furney graduated magna cum laude from the University of Notre Dame and received her doctor of medicine degree with honors from the University of Rochester School of Medicine. After ten years of teaching medical students and residents, she joined a private practice group. In 2000, Furney was diagnosed with multiple sclerosis.